CLINICAL & SPIRITUAL/SOUL CARE PHILOSOPHY

A Minister
A Professor
A Clinical and Spiritual/Biblical Counselor

DR. SABELO SAM MHLANGA

ISBN: 979-8-9899221-0-9 Paperback
ISBN: 979-8-9899221-1-6 Hardback

Independently Published by: Dr Sabelo Sam Mhlanga

Because of the dynamic nature of the Internet, any web addresses or
links contained in this book may have changed since publication and
may no longer be valid. The views expressed in this work are solely
those of the author and do not necessarily reflect the views of the
publisher, and the publisher hereby disclaims any.

TABLE OF CONTENTS

PREFACE

The relational approach to education is fundamental to bringing the reality of theory, knowledge, and wisdom into creating complementary synergies for symbolic rapport and reality. This is an attempt to synchronize Clinical Pastoral Education with the relational education approach to create a sync between the two. In the relational approach to education, radical empathy connects with students and engages them as they intensely, sit for their exams, present their papers, and motivate them to use their abilities as they shape their future. To meet students at their point of need, teachers, lecturers, and professors are obligated to educate the students with passion, empathy, and diligence. The relational approach to education and clinical pastoral education will be explored in the context of Relational Cultural Theory in which the theory advances autonomy, independence, and engagement in growth relationships.

It is in this context that my profound gratitude to the great people at MultiCare Health Systems has shaped my perspectives on clinical education and relational approach to education. The first person who comes to mind is Dr. Annette Gildemann, by then my first preceptor at Auburn Medical Center and now the Clinical and Spiritual Director. Dr. Annette Gildemann was a gentle, caring, and loving mentor. I am indebted to her wisdom and passion for her encouragement to pursue my passion too. The second person who comes to mind who shifted my paradigm of thinking in embracing Emotional Intelligence (EQ) is Rev. Tracey Wilkinson, my supervisor, and Certified Educator. Tracey helped me to break down the walls of concealing my emotions to feel and understand the emotions of my patients as my cultural and traditional norms taught me not to show emotions in public because it is regarded as not representing manhood. I, therefore, dedicate this book to Tracey Wilkinson, my certified Educator.

The other supervisors were Rev. Luz Zemina, and Rabbi Maurice Appelbaum, who mentored and shaped me into understanding to be a good listener and empathic clinical and spiritual care professional.

The preceptors who made a great difference and helped me to be a better clinician and spiritual care professional were James Cornwell at Tacoma General Hospital, Richard Gilbert, and Nicole McKnight. All my peers in Units 1, 2, 3, 4, and 5, were incredible. We launched boats together and had stormy IPR and contentious discussions about hot topics that gave us chills but remained friends. The doctors, nurse manager Angelique Baton, therapists, CNAs, and the HUCS on the 6th floor, where I was placed for a year at Tacoma General Hospital. I was also in Good Samaritan Hospital, Allenmore Hospital, Wellfound Hospital, Mary Bridge Hospital, and Urban Hospitals during my two years as an intern and a resident. Thank you for all your contributions. This book is dedicated to all the people mentioned above and some not mentioned by name.

INTRODUCTION

This project seeks to Integrate the relational approach to education with the intent to develop and cultivate relationships with students in such a way as to bridge education and empathy with the students in a classroom setting. Clinical Pastoral Education is a branch in Chaplaincy settings that offers diverse interdisciplinary multifaith professional health care in hospitals, psychiatric, prisons, police, military business, and clinical fields to offer clinical and spiritual care. It is a program that is set to learn through action-reflection instructional methods which is also a supervised practice. It is designed to prepare students to interact with patients or counselees for effective clinical and spiritual care. This project attempts to take clinical and spiritual care in the hospital setting and apply the techniques, skills, empathy, and emotions to students in education who do not usually experience the practical touch of compassion.

This book discusses the implication and application of spiritual care to students who are academically oriented and inclined to learn head knowledge at learning institutions but learn experiential teaching with their emotions and feelings. This allows students to experience Emotional Intelligence (EQ) in a practical way in which they learn about themselves emotionally and academically. The book concludes with a summary of the philosophy of integration of the Relational Approach to Education and Clinical Pastoral Education.

Chapter One: Relational Approach to Education

The relational Approach to Education is the fundamental essence of integration of education with spiritual care for both students and the staff. It is the epitome of understanding academics and interfacing with relationships. In the original and traditional education system, teachers concentrate on the academic achievement of their students, sometimes ignoring the relational and emotional part of the students. According to Judith V. Jordan and Harriet L. Schwart in their Article, "Radical Empathy in Teaching" propounds, "Relational Cultural Theory has also gained traction in the higher education context as scholars have considered the role of relationships in mentoring and teaching. Studies show that undergraduate students perceived mentoring relationships to be important for success (Beyene et al. 2002) and engagement in mentoring also resulted in higher self-esteem and less loneliness among college-age women (Liang et al. 2002)."[1] They suggest that the relationship is based on mutual empathy. "The pain of social exclusion registers in the same area of the brain (the anterior cingulate) as the pain of physical injury, starvation, or loss of oxygen."[2] In normal academic tradition, education is associated with a concentration on giving information to educate the mind. Radical Empathy in Teaching is a model to shift and integrate with empathy.

Students deserve empathy and cordial relations while being taught. It is in this context that spiritual care needs for students come

---

[1] Judith V. Jordan, and Harriet L. Schwartz, *Radical Empathy in Teaching*, March 2018, (Accessed on   July 23, 2022).
[2] Ibid. p. 25.

alongside teaching, "As we seek to understand and educate our students and assess their work, we experience empathy, "a complex cognitive-affective skill that allows us to 'know' (resonate, feel, sense, cognitively grasp) another person's experience" (Jordan 2010, 103). Empathy is part of the experience of teaching and is often present in our interactions and relationships with students as we (and they) seek to teach and learn the material, understand each other, and move through the course."[3] Showing and understanding students' emotions, challenges and acknowledging their potential, and coming alongside them, give students opportunities to excel. Engagement in relationships is based on mutual empathy that connects students with their teachers and with each other.

From empathy to radical empathy, explores that, "The conventional focus on empathy in educational relationships, like in many hierarchical relationships, is on the professor conveying to a student (or a group of students) some version of, "I sense what you are feeling."[4] As a professor, teacher, instructor, or any kind of leader you are, one must master the skills to relate and interact with students, workers, disciples, or followers. Relational-Cultural Theory is one of the tools that can be employed to bridge relational systems through multicultural and social justice competencies. Dana L. Comstock, propounds, "The key concepts of RCT are perhaps best understood in the context of relational movement, which is the process of moving through connections; through disconnections; and back into new, transformative, and enhanced connections with others... Acquiring this relational awareness is the first step in developing more sophisticated relational capacities that enable one to identify, deconstruct, and resist disconnections and obstacles to

---

[3] Ibid. 25
[4] Judith V. Jordan, and Harriet L. Schwartz, *Radical Empathy in Teaching*, March 2018, (Accessed on   July 23, 2022).

mutual empathy in counseling relationships and the broader culture,"[5] The epitome of connecting with one's students, disciples or those under your supervision is to strike a code of relationship, connecting with the very essence of their being.

In the attempt to connect with your students, disciples, or those under your supervision, they would always be connected, disconnected, and reconnected again. The cycle is inevitable in any relationship. "The Central Relational Paradox theorists have asserted that all individuals have yearnings for connection, belonging, and social inclusion. Despite these yearnings, RCT posits that people commonly demonstrate a paradox in the way they address relational issues in their lives,"[6] Miller and Stiver continue to assert that paradox is activated whenever there is a yearning to connect with people as a strategy to avoid perceived or real risks of hurt, rejection, and other forms of relational disconnection, social exclusion, and marginalization. "Although it is noted that all individuals yearn to connect with other people in authentic, mutually empathic ways, feelings of vulnerability, fear, shame, suspicion, and mistrust make movement into connection difficult."[7] As a leader in one's context, it is fundamental to understand that a relationship with one's subordinates requires moving from head theory to practical relationships to enhance connectivity and rapport with those under one's supervision.

---

[5] Dana L. Comstock, Tonya R. Hammer, Julie Strentzsch, Kristi Cannon, Jacqueline Parsons, and Gustavo Salazar II, Journal of Counseling & Development, Summer 2008, Volume 86, (Accessed April 7, 2023).

[6] Miller & Stiver, 1997, (Accessed April 7, 2023).

[7] Ibid.

Traditional Theories of Psychological Development

Traditional theories of psychological development a theories developed by Linda M. Hartling, Jean Baker Miller, Judith V. Jordan, and Maureen Walker as they laid down the fundamentals of human development citing that, "Growth involves a process of separation from relationship, a process of becoming more independent, autonomous and self-sufficient, and that growth-fostering relationships which are a central human necessity throughout our lives and chronic disconnections which are the source of psychological problems."[8] The thrust of their concepts about psychological development is that it has the power or capacity to produce influence and nature for personal change. In the context of the Central Relational Paradox which purposes every human being yearns to connect, socialize, and interact with others in social spheres and circles to feel belonging and to dispel the fear of disconnection and isolation. Students, disciples, and employees prefer personal connection and belonging. In Chaplaincy, emotional and cognitive connection is fundamental to connecting with patients in the hospital context.

Mutual empathy, care, support, love, and respect are key to fostering relationships to bond and connect with anyone who is under one's supervision. Education in a sense, is not a theory whereby students are given head knowledge only, but education goes beyond head knowledge. May students have emulated and portrayed the characteristics of their professors or teachers in their

[8] Jean Baker Miller Training Institute 2023, (Accessed 10 March 2003).

lives. True education is more of a relationship that will impact the students for the rest of their lives. The symbiotic relationship between the student and the professor/teacher plays a pivotal role in fostering academic excellence. If the student has a good relationship with his/her professor/teacher, he/she excels in his/her class because the love, care, and support of the student are enhanced. The professors/teachers must come down from their horses and relate to their students to promote and develop their students.

Relational approaches to schools or any institutional reforms can fundamentally foster the development of caring relationships among students, teachers, professors, employers, and employees for intellectual, academic, social, and emotional growth. This enhances the sense of belonging, and psychological safety, and promotes rapport that has long-lasting relationships. The caring development approaches aimed at creating a conducive environment for learning can boost relationships among students and teachers. "At its core, relational learning relies on strong relationships between teachers and their students known as a "working alliance." Rather than setting up a dynamic based on power as can be the case in rigid classroom environments, relational learning reimagines the instructor's role as a trusted guide."[9] Research has proven that relational learning benefits students in achieving an emotional, intellectual, and social balance of self-realization and actualization. "By forming positive mentoring relationships with teachers characterized by authenticity, engagement, and empowerment, girls display higher self-esteem and more prosocial behavior."[10] The relational learning approach is more relevant to students of Clinical

---

[9] https://www.oliverianschool.org/why-students-need-relational-learning/, (Accessed June 23, 2023).

[10] Ibid.

and spiritual with their certified educators in the environment of Clinical Pastoral Education (CPE). It is in this context that relational learning approaches can leave a lasting impact in the lives of both the interns and residents in the hospitals as they can take the learning and practice of what they learn in the class and apply it to patients in their respective pains.

Interpersonal Psychotherapy's approach to practice as a clinical profession brings a new perspective and a new dimension to the field. The interpersonal psychotherapy approach has proven to be effective practice if the skills, techniques, and interventions are utilized and practiced. "In highlighting both the covert and overt levels of these relational phenomena and their reciprocity, the interpersonal approach also provides a framework for seamlessly integrating concepts and techniques associated with other treatment approaches to PDs" (Anchin, 1982a, 1982b, 2002; Pincus & Cain, 2008, p. 113. Para. 2). Interpersonal therapy focuses on specific problems of the client and can reduce the symptoms and can create good relationships. It can enhance problem-solving and increase communication skills needed to anchor relationships. These promote interpersonal awareness and learning, resulting in improved relational capacity and symptom reduction. The social learning processes promote both intrapersonal and interpersonal change and enhance communication skills (Anchin, 1982. p. 117. Para. 2).

The emotions and feelings that the client experienced during his/her childhood or with their teachers, parents, relatives, or someone who influenced his/her life, especially negatively, then those feelings are directed to the therapist. The interpersonal Psychology approach to practice presents both benefits as well challenges. The benefits of using the interpersonal psychology approach are that it helps to identify problems expressed in emotions, learning skills to foster good rapport, and focuses on specific problem areas that need to be addressed. It can assist in solving problems, conflicts, and disputes thus improving the therapist's skills of communication by addressing issues such as depression, and anxiety, and being able to administer treatment and symptoms for social adjustment for clients. The other benefit of the interpersonal psychotherapy approach is that it strengthens relationships that can serve as a support network for the benefit of the therapist. "Across all therapeutic modalities, nothing predicts good outcome as reliably as the patient's experience of the therapist as warm, caring, and genuine, and, thus, the patient's experience of being seen, understood and helped," (Safran, J. D., & Muran, J. C. (2000). Interpersonal Psychotherapy approach creates a symbiotic relationship with the client if it is done with empathy and professionalism. It is a type of therapy structured model for treating mental health issues which is timely in the process it improves interpersonal relationships. It is a brief or short-structured therapy that produces immediate results. Transference and countertransference play an important role in the interpersonal psychotherapy approach as has proven to be effective to practice if the skills, techniques, and interventions are utilized and practiced properly.

Interpersonal therapy focuses on specific problems of the client and can reduce the symptoms and can create good relationships. Understanding the client's unconscious impulses, resistance, and transference through intuition, makes the therapist understand unresolved conflicts reflected in the client (Ibid. p. 16. para. 3). It can enhance problem-solving and increase communication skills needed to anchor relationships. These promote interpersonal awareness and learning, resulting in improved relational capacity and symptom reduction. The social learning processes promote both intrapersonal and interpersonal change and enhance communication skills (Anchin, 1982. p. 117. Para. 2). The therapist should be caring, non-judgmental, inspire hope, be able to repair ruptures and find new ways that are better for the clients but sometimes the clients do not see the way out. The client conquered resistance and admitted the instinctual and emotional complexes that have the flashbacks from his past into his consciousness, impeded by the unexpected phenomenon of transference. The interpersonal Psychotherapy approach is very fundamental in assessing, evaluating, assigning clients with DSM criteria, and applying practical treatment.

Sigmund Freud developed the concept of countertransference to refer to a situation in which the psychologist's emotions, unconsciously, are transferred and influenced by a person in therapy, and the reaction by the psychologist is called countertransference (Good-Therapy, 2007). www.goodtherapy.org). Freud continues to hold on saying that both ego and shadow are accepted as essential counterparts in psychic wholeness (Ibid. 30. para. 2).

Professional psychology has started to shift toward a competent-based model of training in recent decades. There have been some significant made towards competencies in professional psychology. Donovan, R. A. and Ponce, A. N., (2009). The shift to the culture of a competence-based model ushers in a new dimension into addressing public trust and protection of the citizen. Donovan and Ponce assert, "Other potential benefits include: a more flexible training model based on the trainees' needs and progress toward established goals… improved connections between graduate training and the skills needed to practice as a psychologist, anticipating likely increased competency requirements by federal and state regulatory bodies… and keeping pace with other health care professions …" Donovan, R. A., and Ponce, A. N., (2009). p. 546. This new shift brings with it new and high anticipation and zeal to the psychological fraternity. The evolution to change the old model and the contribution and benefits of competence-based education will forever change the perspective and the paradigm of thinking. Donovan and Ponce reiterate the fact that, "the foundational competencies address the 'knowledge, skills, attitudes, and values' psychologists need in their professional roles… and the functional competencies address the functions psychologists perform," (para. 2), to add value and create relationships between the clinical psychologists and the patients. The competency-based education movement for the training of professional psychologists contributes a benchmark in professional psychology in that it outlines the core foundational and functional competencies in three levels of professional development i.e., readiness practicum, internship, and entry to practice, (Fouad, Nadya. A., Grus, Catharine. L., Hatcher, Robert. L., Kaslow Nadine. J., Hutchings, P. S., Madison, M. B. Crossman, R. E., email, 2009).

The role and the importance of relationship competency to the practice of professional psychology is by design, aimed at developing relationships with the client to gain trust and mutual understanding between the clinician and the patients. "The path broadens through the development of trust, safety, and understanding as the relationship develops," Capuzzi, D., and Stauffer D. M., (2016). The relationship competency to professional psychology has gained popularity in recent decades and Kaslow points out the eight elements: "Eight of the 10 workgroups were formed around competency domains: (a) ethical and legal issues, (b) individual and cultural diversity, (c) scientific foundations and research, (d) psychological assessment, (e) intervention, (f) consultation and interprofessional collaboration, (g) supervision, and (h) professional development," Kaslow, Nadine J. (2004). To develop relationships with your clients/patients, the clinician must develop and foster a good rapport with them. The relationship competency for professional psychology demands that nowadays. Understanding cultural diversity and cultural values, religions, and ethical and legal issues of an organization one works with cultivates and develops relationships. This includes the relationship with the staff one works with, the boards, the management, and the institution.

Chapter Two: Integration of Relational Approach to Clinical Pastoral Education

In this chapter, I will quote, and reference Clinical Pastoral Education offered by MultiCare Healthy Systems at Good Samaritan and Tacoma General Hospitals which offer this program. In the same vein, I acquired my five (5) Units as an intern and a resident, respectively. I had extensive training with my CPE-certified educators, Rabbi Maurice Appelbaum, Rev. Luz Zemina, and Rev. Tracey Wilkinson, and of course, the Spiritual Director, Dr. Annette Gildemann. I owe them great respect and honor for their training and inspiration, genius, and for being proactive in their conduct and professionalism. "Good Samaritan was established in January 1952 when the Lutheran Home and Welfare Society assumed management of Puyallup General Hospital at the request of the doctors who owned that facility. Clinical Pastoral Education began at Good Samaritan Hospital in 1972, providing clinical education programs for local clergy and seminarians from around the country. The Good Samaritan CPE program was a satellite of the CPE program at Swedish Medical Center, Seattle, WA. MultiCare Good Samaritan Hospital is accredited to offer Level I and Level II ACPE Certified CPE™ by the Association for Clinical Pastoral Education," (Student Handbook, 2022-2023).

CPE is an action/reflection professional educational experience. As an intern or a resident, you are authorized to visit clients/patients and their families as a Spiritual Care Professional and to be as informed of their physical, spiritual, emotional, psychological, and sociological situation as the policies of institutions allow.

You are authorized to write materials beneficial to your educational process based on visits made under the overall supervision of an assigned ACPE Certified Educator and the on-site consultation of a liaison/mentor assigned by the institution(s) in which your visit occurs. Confidentiality is basic to your professional role, and any communication, regarding patients outside our professional treatment and/or CPE process is prohibited, except as required for the safety of clients/patients, families, or others, (Student Handbook, 2022-2023). It is a violation of confidentiality and hospital protocol to publish information on social computing platforms that are related to patient health information.

Clinical Pastoral Education's thrust is to foster pastoral/spiritual care as an important component of the healing process. As a clinical and spiritual professional, you are angled to provide physical, emotional, and spiritual care to patients according to their wishes and needs. It is patient-centered, not clinician-centered. The CPE program is run through the Spiritual Care Department which provides excellent spiritual care to hospitals. The care focuses on the patients, their families, and the staff.

Clinical Pastoral Education (CPE) is experiential theological education that is designed to increase self-awareness and to develop and sharpen the student's ability to provide spiritual care for patients, families, and staff. "Clinical Pastoral Education (CPE) began in 1925 as a form of theological education that takes place not exclusively in academic classrooms, but also in clinical settings where ministry is being practiced. CPE is offered in many kinds of settings: in hospitals and health care including university, children's, and veterans' facilities; in hospices; in psychiatric and community care facilities; in workplace settings; in geriatric and rehabilitation centers; and congregational and parish-based settings."[11] The program is the training of compassionate presence and grounded in the spiritual and soul care of patients and clients. Clinical Pastoral Education prepares one as a spiritual, vocational, and professional clinician. It is an interfaith program that prepares an individual to be able to be equipped to listen, be present, to come alongside patients. It provides you with integrated, interfaith, and applied theology education. CPE is an approved corporate clinical training and the four entities, Institute of Pastoral Care, Lutheran Advisory Council, Southern Baptist for Clinical Pastoral Education, and Association for Clinical Pastoral Education emerged into the Association for Clinical Pastoral Education. "The organization has three commissions: Standards, Accreditation of Centers, and Certification of Supervisors of clinical pastoral education Since 1969 it has been on the Federal Government's Department of Education's Commissioner's list of nationally recognized accrediting agencies/associations in the field of clinical pastoral education."[12]

The background or theory of Clinical Pastoral Education draws its strength and purpose, from other educational systems, from the fact that " An underpinning theory of education that structures clinical pastoral education is the "Action-Reflection" mode of learning. CPE students typically compose "verbatims" of their pastoral care encounters in which they are invited to reflect upon what occurred and draw insight from these reflections that can be implemented in future pastoral care events."[13] Action reflection, emotional intelligence, connection, disconnection, and reconnection

---

[11] https://ucsfspiritualcare.org/history, (Accessed August 3, 2023).

[12] Ibid.

[13] Ibid.

again, are the main ballgame of the CPE. In the same vein, empathy, compassion, love, and care are the gist of the characteristics of Clinical Pastoral Education.

Clinical Pastoral Education is designed and has a detailed program to equip students to administer their expertise to patients and clients for clinical and spiritual care. The following is the general curriculum of CPE as outlined by the Institute for Clinical Pastoral Training:

- 100 hours of didactic lectures offered live and via interactive distance learning.
- Weekly Reflection Reports which depict significant experiences with patients and thoughts.
- Case Studies that outline interactions with patients or counselees.
- Weekly one-on-one Coaching/Supervisory Sessions with experienced CPE Supervisors. The students receive personalized instruction, guidance, and mentoring.
- Students participate in interactive Peer Reviews where they discuss their work and the work conducted by their classmates. Peer review in the CPE program provides opportunities for students to expand their perspectives and collaborate with interdisciplinary teams.
- CPE students partake in 300 hours of supervised Clinical Training at their current place of ministry or any number of settings including but not limited to; hospitals, hospice houses, corporate settings, prison systems, skilled nursing facilities, nursing homes, assisted living facilities, and community organizations.
- Full-Time: A full-time unit is 12 weeks long and includes at least 300 hours of direct clinical contact hours with designated

clientele or patients and 100 hours of lecture and peer review with a group of not less than two peers. The student must be engaged in a clinical ministry setting no less than 25 hours per week.

- Part Time: A part-time unit is 24 weeks long and includes at least 300 hours of direct clinical contact hours with designated clientele or patients and 100 hours of lecture and peer review with a group of not less than two peers. The student must be engaged in a clinical ministry setting no less than 12.5 hours per week.[14]

Clinical pastoral education (CPE) is a combination of professional education and firsthand experience, providing spiritual care to patients, families, and staff members in multi-faith clinical settings. Clinical Pastoral Education has a different setting than Pastoral Theology. It is not in the definition and philosophy of "Pastoring" per sei, but CPE philosophy is patient-centered not clinician-centered. The clinician gives all the attention, listening, and focus to the patient, coming alongside him/her. It is not like the usual phenomenon of a pastor running the show. Clinical Pastoral is an accredited form of spiritual care education that is linked to the Association for Clinical Pastoral Education (ACPE). "Reflection on clinical experiences helps students become more self-aware, develop, and increase their listening skills, spiritual assessment skills, and their competence in providing meaningful interventions. Through this transformative process, students find and claim their pastoral identity and authority."[15]

---

[14] https://www.icpt.edu/what-is-cpe.html, (Accessed August 12, 2023).

[15] https://college.mayo.edu/academics/health-sciences-education/clinical-pastoral-education-residency-minnesota/curriculum/, (Accessed August 21, 2023).

CPE is designed to call oneself to realize and recognize who you are, to accept your identity, embrace both your weaknesses and strengths, and be able to feel for others and empathize, therefore, with their situations and circumstances. This enhances one's ability to dialogue with one's spiritual heritage and behavioral sciences. In the process, it provides an opportunity to integrate personal and professional growth to be a better clinician to transform the educational experience.

The scope of Clinical Pastoral Education derives its essence from living human documents which are caregiving, self-care, and the study of ourselves as individuals and as a people. It focuses on individual development and the skills of spiritual caregivers to provide holistic health care and spiritual care to patients or clients in any given institution. The students of Clinical Spiritual Education are given space to explore their beliefs and values as part of the learning process to produce the best version of themselves. "The primary goal of CPE is to enhance the personal and professional development of the student as a spiritual caregiver. The program is designed to provide students with opportunities for self-reflection and self-awareness and to develop pastoral skills such as active listening, empathetic communication, and ethical decision-making. CPE programs involve supervised clinical work with patients and families and regular group and individual supervision with a certified supervisor."[16]

The integration of a relational approach to clinical pastoral education seeks to explore the relationships between the students, certified educators, and staff with mutual respect. The relationship approach to education enhances good rapport between the students

---

[16] https://www.davidfleenor.org/post/what-is-clinical-pastoral-education, (Accessed September 26, 2023).

and the teacher/professor. It means students and teachers/professors develop good and sound relationships that create a safe environment for education. In the same vein the educators, interns, and residents in a hospital setting can foster connection and develop mutual, respect and dignity if they relate well. Education is an invitation to personal growth through a transaction of knowledge between the teacher/professor and students. Relationship learning is an approach is a supportive relationship that supports shared learning experiences. "At its core, relational learning relies on strong relationships between teachers and their students known as a "working alliance." Rather than setting up a dynamic based on power as can be the case in rigid classroom environments, relational learning reimagines the instructor's role as a trusted guide. While instructors in more traditional settings can certainly function as guides and can form deep connections with students, truly relational learning makes the working alliance central to the broader educational experience."[17]

The integration of a relational approach informs clinical pastoral education to act as co-joins to foster rapport among the students, staff, patients, and certified educators allowing a holistic approach to both physical and spiritual care. The genuine interaction between theory and practice enhances the skills and expertise of the staff and the students as they discharge their services. One of the ways to consolidate and solidify relationships.

---

[17] https://www.oliverianschool.org/why-students-need-relational-learning/ (Accessed October 6, 2023).

Chapter Three: A Minister

To be a Minister/Pastor is a calling from God. It is confirmed by the call of Jeremiah (Jeremiah 1:5, CSB). God declared that he chose Jeremiah before he was formed in the womb, set apart before he was born, and appointed him to be a prophet to the nations. God points out the three fundamental verbs about the calling of the prophet Jeremiah: **formed, set apart**, and **appointed.** Before God formed Jeremiah in the womb, he knew him. It means that before the formation of a person in the womb, the person exists in the bosom of God, outside matter. It means God knew him before the foundation of the world. When a person is conceived in the womb, the person is known by God, and it means the person existed outside the womb. God knows the person before his/her existence in the flesh. God knits the person in the womb, in a mystical way, and a miraculous way. He then inhales his own Spirit and then the matter becomes a living being (Genesis 2:7, NIV). God calls certain people and then he narrates how the person becomes a being and then he sets them apart for special services. God knows about each of us.

The second, aspect is that when someone has been conceived and has become a matter, a human being, God sets him/her apart for a special service. Set apart means being sanctified, which means to be separated. God does not call you without tracing your origin, the task that he has called you to do, and then informing you of his provision, protection, and security. When God sanctifies you, he has a special task that he wants you to accomplish, no other person could do. In (Ephesians 4:11-13, CSB), God specifies the ministry or tasks of those who are called into the ministry, "And himself gave some to be apostles, some prophets, some evangelists, some pastors, and teachers, equipping the saints for the work of ministry, to build up the body of Christ, until we all reach unity in the faith and the knowledge of God's Son, growing into maturity with a stature measured by Christ's fullness." When God set you apart for a specific mission, Paul outlined them to the church. When God sets you apart for the special service, as an apostle, a prophet, an evangelist, a pastor, or a teacher, he wants to fulfill all these five-fold ministries that are designed to equip the church.

The third aspect is the appointment to a specific place in terms of geographical areas in the world. With a special gift that God gives his servants, he sees it fit for a particular individual to relocate to a specific area. For example, God commissioned Jonah to go to Ninevah for a special and specific mission for the city to repent for their sins. "The word of the Lord came to Jonah's son of Amittai: Get up! Go to the great city of Ninevah and preach against it because their evil has come up before me," (Jonah 1:1, CSB). God wanted Jonah to preach the gospel to the city of Ninevah. There are two things I want to highlight about being created by God, knowing you before he formed you in the womb, setting you apart for a special and specific task, and being appointed to a specific geographic city, nation, or continent. However, God gives us the choice to agree to the call or to refuse but ultimately, God's will prevail regardless of your willingness or not. Jonah is a good example of being known by God before existence in the flesh, set apart after being born for a special and specific and then he was appointed to preach to Ninevah.

In that context, two callings should be brought to the right perspective. The first calling is when God knows you before you formed in the womb not by one's choice but by God's choice. The second calling is when you are born and set apart and appointed for the task and you respond positively or negatively. Some people are called into the ministry when they are young, and they respond to the call, but others resist the call and keep on postponing until they respond when they are advanced in age. One example of the person who was called into the ministry was Moses, who was eighty years old, called to deliver the people of God, from Egypt, (Exodus 7:7, CSB). Moses gave excuses to God when he commissioned him to go and deliver the children of Israel. "But Moses said to God, 'Who am I, that I should go to Pharoah and bring the Israelites out of Egypt... (Exodus 3:11, CSB). He also gave an excuse to God, explaining that he cannot speak well or stutter, (Exodus 4:10-12, CSB). In the New Testament, Jesus Christ called his 12 disciples through prayer, "One of those days Jesus went out to a mountainside to pray and spent the night praying to God. When morning came, he called his disciples to him and chose twelve of them, whom he also designated apostles," (Luke 6:12-13, NIV).

The question one may ask is, how were you called to the ministry? Did you respond to the call as a minister, right away or did you resist the call first and respond later? What were the signs to confirm and affirm that God was calling you into the ministry? How has been the ministry since you responded to the call? How have your wife and children been involved in the ministry? Are there any challenges you have faced or are you facing in the ministry? These are some of the questions I will explore and answer in this chapter.

In 1985, there was a missionary, Jerald Haadsma who visited our school to show films to all interested students. He came with Rev. Jealous Manyumbu who was a local Pastor at West Nicholson, pastoring African Evangelical Church. They used to come every Sunday afternoon around 6:00 pm. It was good entertainment for many students because we had no entertainment except soccer on weekends. Showing films was important and there were Christian films only and there were no options. We all loved Sunday's entertainment. Many of us became devoted Christians and Rev. Jealous Manyumbu and Jerald Haadsma, a missionary from Grand Rapids in USA, were now leading the interdenominational school church. Jerald's wife Florence Haadsma was always coming with her husband for the new ministry which they had started in the school. They organized to start a church at the school because before showing the films, Rev. J. Manyumbu and J. Haadsma would preach the gospel to the students for repentance and many students repented. They later changed the church services to 3:00 pm at school and we got involved in inviting students to come to church. It was at this time in 1985 that I rededicated my life to Christ, and I repented from all my sins, and I asked Christ to forgive me. After Jesus' film was shown, depicting his gruesome slogging, and painful death, it dawned on me that Christ is my Savior. When Haadsma explained salvation, justification, sanctification, and glorification, and also quoted some verses from the Bible such as "For all have sinned and come short of the glory of God," (Romans 3:23, NIV), "If you declare with your mouth, 'Jesus is Lord,' and believe in your heart that God raised him from the dead, you will be saved," (Romans 10:9, NIV). It became clear to me that Jesus is the Savior of the world. I was thoroughly convicted and convinced that for sure I needed Jesus in my life.

In November 1985, I sat for my junior certificate examination in Form Two and that's when I got baptized also at West Nicholson by Jerald Haadsma with many other students. In 1986, Jerald Haadsma and Rev. Jealous Manyumbu trusted me and gave me the authority to keep the film equipment in my dormitory for them for the following Sunday. Meanwhile, I was elected as the chairman of Scripture Union, the chairman of the interdenominational church, and the Impala dormitory prefect. I used to take the Christian students out in the rivers and jungle to pray and fast, (*Enhlane*). Austin Mabhena and Godfrey Ngwenya were part of the group I used to lead and pray with them. People were now calling me a Pastor. I drew more respect from students, teachers, and school staff because of my Christian beliefs, conviction, and character. I had close friends who were not Christians such as Ndondela, and Alfa Ncube, and many who overheard that there was a conspiracy plot to attack me by some of the students because of my popularity at the school and of my Christian life. As a Christian group, we went out of school in the jungle as Christians to pray and fast for my protection from evil during the weekends and that rumor just dispelled in the thick air. We saw the hand of God at work and His protection. Jerald Haadsma enrolled me and others in Bible Correspondence School courses and I completed all the levels required to graduate with a diploma. Mr. Haadsma was very impressed with my determination and hard work. He advised me that when I completed my school, I should consider going to Bible College to study Theology, at Theological College of Zimbabwe in Bulawayo.

I used to go to Scripture Union camps during the school breaks. In August school break in 1986, I went to a Scripture Union camp at Matopo Hills, in South of Bulawayo. During the camp, at break time, I picked up a pamphlet which was written about the dilemma of Sarah and Abraham who did not have a promised son, at their advanced ages, Sarah at 90 or 91 years old and Abraham was 100 years old. The pamphlet continued to say that if you know a neighbor, a sister, or an aunt who cannot have children, you must pray for them. Maybe God can open their wombs. I took it to heart. One of my sisters, Senzeni Khatha, was happily married to Amos

Maseko but she always had multiple miscarriages at four or five months pregnant. I earnestly asked God to help my sister to have at least one child. I vowed to God that if God would give my sister Senzeni and Amos Maseko a child, I would serve Him for the rest of my life. God honored my prayer for my sister and my brother-in-law, they had a handsome baby boy in 1987 and they named him Mandlenkosi (The Power of God). I kept my vow in my heart. I did tell them that I had prayed for them to have a child, but they did not understand it. But it was my secret with my God, and I kept the vow and treasured it in my heart.

My final years at J. Z. High School were a great challenge as I was busy preparing for examinations. I was also a student leader, and the Vice President of the Student Union, and Frank Sibanda was the President. I knew where to go when I faced difficulties in decision-making and facing life challenges, to Christ. My time at J. Z. High School was coming to an end and I was to seek the face of the Lord and ask for His direction for my future. I decided to pray and fast for seven days for my future career and profession. I had decided on two things for my life. My supplication to God was that if God could direct me to be a Minister/Pastor. That was my priority and my first call. My second priority was that if God was not calling me to a full-time ministry, I would want to be a businessman, to support the church at large with my businesses. Those were the two requests that were submitted to the Lord before I wrote my examinations in November 1987. I fasted for seven days and pleaded with the Lord to show me the way. After classes, I would go into the jungle to fast the whole day and I would break with dinner for seven days. After seven days, I did not hear any answers from the Lord. I took my exams and waited for the results at home. While I was waiting for my examination results at home, waiting for

God's answer and pondering what I would do next. Come January 1988, I enrolled in Business Courses at Zimbabwe Commercial College in downtown, Bulawayo. I enrolled to study Business and Office Practice, preparing to start a business when I completed my studies, and I took it as a confirmation that God had wanted me to do that as he did not confirm the calling of being a Pastor. My home was at Pumula North, but I wanted to be closer to Bulawayo downtown for a walking distance to the College as I did not have money to get to the buses every day. So, I asked my uncle Moses' son who had a house in Makhokhoba Township very close to downtown where the college was. I lived with him for a year studying Business. He graciously agreed to take me in. I lived with him with his other cousin, Christian Nkabinde, and his elder brother and his wife. We had a very good relationship with Christian Nkabinde and his brother. I used to wake up early in the morning and walk about two to three kilometers to college. The government paid for my education through a scholarship that we were granted as returnees. The scholarship covered books and a small stipend but not accommodation.

While I was studying my Business and Office Practice, God spoke to me strongly that this was not where I was supposed to be. There was a College at Lobengula Street called Theological College of Zimbabwe where most of my friends I was at J. Z. High School and George Silundika High School, were studying Theology. Some of my friends heard that I was studying Business and Office Practice courses at Zimbabwe Commercial College. They visited me and they told me that they were studying theology at Theological College of Zimbabwe. I told them that God had not called me yet and I was following my second passion. I continued my studies for the whole of 1988 at Zimbabwe Commercial College. At the end of the year in 1988, God convicted me so strongly that I had to go to Theological College, but I did not want to just jump on it without His confirmation. I was intending to continue with my course in Business Studies and Office Practice. In March 1989 during the night, I heard a voice calling me. I woke up and asked my mother if she was calling me, but she said that she had not called me. I went back to sleep. The same voice called me for the second time, and I asked my mother if she had called me, but she said that she had not called me. I was now wondering who the person who was calling me, audibly, was at midnight. The third time, the voice called me again and this time I remembered Samuel who was called by God three times, (I Samuel 3:10, NKJV). I started praying and telling God that I was accepting the call to serve Him. I remembered the vow I had made when I was praying for sister Senzeni and her husband, Amos Maseko who did not have a child with several miscarriages finally, God gave them a son, Mandlenkosi, and the vow that I had made with God if He would answer my prayer, He did. I was now on board to go to Theological College of Zimbabwe. When the schools opened in January, I still went back to pursue Business Studies and Office Practice although I had agreed with God to go to a Theological College to study Theology, but the question was how. The government was not going to pay for any religious carrier. If one took that route, it was the end of government scholarships.

While I was in the class, I heard that there was someone who was calling me outside. I got out and who did I saw, it was Newman Kolobe, an old friend of mine at George Silundika High School who was a student evangelist at the school. Newman Kolobe did not mince his words but told me that I was not in the right place at that College. I explained to him that I was waiting for God to provide for the school fees. He told me to go to the Theological College to talk to President Molly. After class, I went to Theological College of Zimbabwe and when a group of students saw me, especially those who knew me, they welcomed me and directed me to Molly, the Principal of the Theological College of Zimbabwe. In his office, he asked me about my calling to the ministry. I did not know that Rev. Jealousy Manyumbu and Jerald Haasdma had mentioned my name to him long before. Within 30 minutes, I was admitted to Theological College of Zimbabwe to study Theology, and I was granted a full scholarship for three years from 1989 to 1991. The ways of the Lord are different from our ways. I was told to go and get my belongings and start my studies in August 1989.

When I told my mother and my siblings that I was going to Theological College of Zimbabwe in Bulawayo and that I would be boarding. They were very happy and thrilled for me the opportunity was given. They told me that they knew that I would eventually train as a Minister as my character and my passion were evident. It was good for me too to be in a boarding school again and pursue my studies. I was granted a full scholarship for tuition, boarding, and living expenses. I was glad to meet once again with Austin Mabhena whom I had led to go to church while we were students at J. Z. High School and that he was now being trained as a minister of the Gospel. My lecturers were impressive, such as Dr. Burgess, Dr. Heaton, Jenny Smith, Rev. Mabhena, and many others. As I got assimilated into the TCZ system, I was appointed to be an Assistant Librarian with Adamson Nyoni and Jenny Smith was the senior Librarian and a Lecturer as well. We used to have shifts with Adamson Nyoni and when he graduated, I became a Librarian with Jenny Smith helping me, but she was concentrating more as a lecturer. TCZ was looking for a librarian to fill the position as a full-time librarian.

Pursuing my studies at the Theological College of Zimbabwe (TCZ) was a blessing. I used to earn my salary as a Librarian and the stipend that the college used to give us.

I ministered to four churches, City United Baptist Church, Sakubva United Baptist Church, Dangamvura United Baptist Church, Chikanga United Baptist Church, and other minor preaching points in Mutare City and the surrounding peri-auburn areas. I preached to these churches in rotation, once a month, for each church. I did counsel for the church members. I organized a mass wedding for 30 couples who were members of the four churches who were married but did not have their weddings. Rev. Guest Myambo helped me to counsel the couple and I asked Dr. Bishop Joshua Dhube to officiate the mass weddings because I was not yet licensed to officiate the weddings. It was a happy day for the couples and their families on the wedding day. I had District youths from the four churches who were very committed to evangelism outreach, and I used to organize evangelism outreaches. The places we used to have evangelism outreach were Imbeza, Odzi, and Burma Valley. One incident that caught the eyes of many youths about the belief and reality that we are not fighting against the flesh and blood but against principalities, against dark forces in the heavenly places, as Apostle Paul alludes in (Eph. 6:12, NIV). During the outer call, many people came forward with their charms, talismans, ritual clothes, and ornaments as they wanted to trust in Jesus alone and surrender what they used to believe in. It was a scary service as many local people went home to collect their secret ornaments, charms dedicated to the devil. They threw their items in the front and the heap grew up slowly until it was huge. One woman came to me to hand over something in her hand, a charm. She said that the charm was for her luck and protecting her life and she had depended on it for many years, but she wanted to depend on Christ alone. I took it in my hand, and I remember it was dark with a few lambs around. When I stretched my hand toward her to receive the charm, the charm was breathing. It was wrapped in cloth, black and greasy cloth, and breathing as if it had a heartbeat. I held it in my hands while I was leading people to dedicate their lives to Jesus. After praying with the people, and ending the service, I took some of the few youths outside the building to a youth advisor Mr. E. Myambo, who was also one of the prominent elders of Sakubva UBC. We made some fire to burn the charms, the ornaments, the clothes dedicated to ancestral spirits, and the charm that the woman had given me and placed on the hand.

As I was about to throw the charm from my hand into the fire, Mr. E. Myambo advised me that I should not burn it; instead, we should dig a hole and bury it. He told me about an incident that was experienced by another Pastor who burnt such kinds of stuff, the ornaments, and the charms in which the flames of fire lipped on his body and burnt him entirely. So, he feared for me, and he wanted to protect me from any dangers. He was genuine however, I believed God would protect me from such kinds of incidents. I threw the breathing charm into the fire too and everything was burnt to ashes. After disciplining the woman with others, I baptized her in Sakubva UBC together with others who had confessed Jesus as Lord and Savior. Christ's name was exalted in Burma Valley UBC preaching point. We used to organize many evangelistic outreaches in Burma Valley. We would play soccer with the local teams to witness them during the games and invite them to the evening programs in their places of gathering. The Lord was with us, and He gave us the passion to witness Him. The youths were the vehicle in which my ministry in the Mutare district flourished. I connected well with the youth because I was a youth too although I was a Pastor. I also connected well with all the members of the four churches as I was a Pastor regardless of age. It was three fruitful years of ministry in Mutare City before I left to go and further my studies at Africa University in Mutare.

In 2008, I relocated with my family to further my studies in the USA in Grand Rapids, Michigan. I was studying master's in theology in a Seminary. After graduating in May 2010, we moved to Louisville, Kentucky to further my Doctorate. After completing my Doctorate, I was hired by North American Mission Board, and Send Network as a Church Planter/Missionary. We started the Bread of Life International Fellowship (BOLIF) in Kent, Washington. I have been a minister of this church since 2016. We have opened another branch in Tacoma, Washington. Pastoring is my passion and a calling, to plant churches. We have evangelism outreach, basketball camps, block parties, and school outreach through school supplies to the local schools. We also had a program for homeless outreach before Covid-19 came. I planted a church in London, United Kingdom in 2005 and it is still growing even today. In 2023, I planted a church, our home church, United Baptist Church USA/Canada. We launched it on August 27, 2023, and the President of United Baptist Church, Bishop Austin Mabhena came from Zimbabwe to launch it. Glory be to God!!

Chapter Four: A Professor

The years at Africa University were fruitful and I will always cherish them and be grateful to the Theology Faculty, Faculty of Education, and the Africa University administration.

After graduation, what was next? I had already decided that I would go for teaching for a while before I returned to Pastoring because Pastoring was my calling while teaching was my profession. My wife, Judith, and I were now preparing to relocate to Bulawayo, my home city from Mutare. We had lived in Mutare for almost ten years, and it was time for us to go and live in my home city in Bulawayo. I graduated on July 1, 2000, and I went to Bulawayo to look for a teaching position. My wife was still teaching at Mutsvangwa High School, and we hoped that after securing the teaching position, my wife Judith would get a transfer letter and we would teach at the same school, God willing, in Bulawayo. We prayed about God's guidance. The schools were to open in early September 2000. I wanted to beat that time so that by the beginning of the term, September to December, I would have secured a teaching position. We planned that we would move to Bulawayo after I got a teaching position in Bulawayo. I went to Bulawayo and the following day; I went to the Ministry of Education Recruiting Head Office which was located at the Main Post Office by then. I got into their office and met with the education recruiting officer who told me that I could not get any teaching position in the Bulawayo district or peri-urban, it was impossible because they were a list of senior teachers who were waiting to transfer to Bulawayo City and for me as a new teacher, I should first be deployed to the rural schools before applying for a teaching position in Bulawayo City. They told me that that was the procedure.

There were two officers in the office and when they looked at my certificates, they were very impressed with my bachelor's degree certificate from African University. They looked at my transcript and saw that my major was Divinity, and my minor was Education in History. One of them took me to the other office to check on the openings. They started talking to each other and one of them said that there was an opening at Pumula East Secondary School. They started arguing that as a new teacher, according to the policy, I could not start teaching in the City when thousands of teachers had been waiting to transfer to come to teach in Bulawayo City and they could not violate that policy. It would be detrimental to their responsibility and the breach of the Ministry of Education policy. They went to another office to check, and they left me in their office. After thirty minutes, they came back and told me that they were going to give me a letter to the Headmaster/Principal of Pumula East Secondary School to take the open History teaching position. I could see the favor of God upon me, no doubt about that, because just the fact that they agreed to let me go with the letter to the Headmaster/Principal of Pumula East Secondary School, was not something unheard of.

I took the letter to the Headmaster/Principal of Pumula East Secondary School and when I got there, I got into the Headmaster/Principal's office. The Recruiting Education Officers from the Ministry of Education had called the Headmaster/Principal and told him that I was on the way to fill the teaching position of History. He was pleased to offer me that History teaching position at the school. I was amazed at how God directed the whole process so easily and without any delays. It was as if the position was kept for me with great favor. The Headmaster/Principal was so friendly, and he took me to the classes I would be teaching when the school opened in a few weeks. He showed me my class and the office. I was so excited to start my teaching career in my home city, Bulawayo. I thanked God and praised Him for His mercy and His intervention at an appropriate time. I went back to Mutare and told my wife what had happened, and the way God had opened the doors for me to teach in the City of Kings and Queens, Bulawayo. It was school break at that time, and we started packing to move to Bulawayo.

While I had gone to Bulawayo, my wife told me that one of the members of the National Committee, Mr. Cephas Ngarinvhume had come while I was away and was sent by the Head Office of United Baptist Church to ask me to go and teach at Rusitu Bible College as a lecturer. What a surprise and the turn of events! He had told my wife, Judith that he would come again to see and talk to me about asking me to be a lecturer at Rusitu Bible College. I thought to myself that God is not the God of confusion. He could not open two doors at the same time. Mr. Cephas Ngarivhume and the Principal of Rusitu Bible College, Rev. Timothy Barrow, eventually, came and told me that they had been sent by the National Committee from the Head Office and Dr. Bishop Joshua Dhube to ask me to go and be a lecturer at the Bible College. They presented me with a crisis Rev. Tim Barrow, the Principal of Rusitu Bible School, was taking another position full-time at Serving in Missions, (SIM) and they needed me to bridge the gap while waiting for the incoming new Principal, Rev. Onias Tapera to take over from Rev. Tim. Barrow. Rev. O. Tapera was to come some few months to come but he was still in Denver, Colorado. He had just completed his master's in divinity from the Seminary. So, my task was to be a lecturer at Rusitu Bible College and to be an interim person between outgoing, Rev. Tim Barrow who was leaving for a new position in Serving in Missions (SIM), and incoming Principal, Rev. Onias Tapera from the USA.

It was the shock of my life how to manage the two dilemmas in front of me, to be honest. Whom do I pledge my allegiance to, the Ministry of Education or the Church, to serve as a lecturer? To put it simply, to be a Lecturer at a College or to be a Teacher at a High School? Which one would you choose if it were you? Well, it was a dilemma for me for a while. Teaching was a good job offer with a reliable salary every month. I had secured a teaching position in the city of Bulawayo, my own home in which so many teachers had waited for five or ten years to get a teaching position in the city of Bulawayo. I had just got a teaching position without any struggle at all. The Lecturers were the same as the Pastors who were struggling to get decent pay or salary every month. Now I was left with two choices, to bend to a secular job or to stretch to God's work. I asked them to give us a few days to ponder and pray about the request. We discussed and prayed about the right decision to make with my wife, Judith. Finally, God helped us to choose His work rather than the secular job although there were some greener pastures in the secular job, I decided to suffer with the people of God rather than enjoy the pleasures of this world for a season. It was painful to call the Pumula East Secondary School Headmaster/Principal to tell him what had transpired and that I was no longer coming to join his teaching staff in September 2000. The headmaster was very disappointed about my decision because he was looking forward to working with me and he said that he was thrilled to introduce me to his teaching staff and to the students when schools opened and to restart again in looking for a history teacher.

I finally accepted the position to be a lecturer at Rusitu Bible College and to function as an interim person between Rev. Tim. Barrow and Rev. Onias Tapera who was anticipated to resume Principalship at Rusitu Bible College. We packed our furniture and belongings to move to Rusitu Bible College. After the interviews and all the procedures necessary, we moved to Rusitu Bible College. "In their hearts, humans plan their course, but the Lord establishes their steps," (Proverbs 16:9, NIV). Rev. Tim Barrow moved our furniture to Rusitu with his truck. My wife was still a teacher at Mutsvangwa Secondary School when I moved to Rusitu Bible College. It did not take long before my wife was given a teaching position at Rusitu High School, per our request. It was a great benefit for the first time to live together with my wife under one roof. It was in August 2000 that we arrived at Rusitu Bible College. Our second child, a daughter, was born in September 2000 after we had settled in Rusitu.

I found Rodney Kastner and Rev. Masango Matimura who were the lecturers/professors, and I took over some of the necessary positions to put things in order as Rev. Tim Barrow exited and he showed me what to do before Rev. Onias Tapera came. I was given the mandate to be an interim person while waiting for Rev. Onias Tapera to come from the USA. Judith Khumbula was the College Secretary. Rusitu Bible College started in 1963 with only one student but it has grown steadily now. The College gets its sponsorship from the churches and well-wishers for the running of the College and for paying the lecturers although their salaries come directly from the United Baptist Church Head Office. I was now in charge of the College, awaiting the coming of Rev. Onias Tapera and it did not take long before he arrived with his family. I showed him what Rev. Tim Barrow had shown me to show the new Principal. I was the lecturer and the Dean of Students.

We had great students from different churches who sent their students for theological training and to be equipped for ministry, with United Baptist Church students being the majority always. We became so close with Rev. Tapera, Rev. Masango Matimura, and Rev. Timothy Myambo who later joined us as a lecturer and Rev. Onias Tapera became the College Principal. We had a good community of friends. Rev. Timothy Myambo became a part-time Pastor for our Mission Station, Rusitu United Baptist Church. He organized family fellowships in the mission in which we would gather every Saturday and bring potluck for each family to share. It was a good time to be close to families within the Mission Station in the community. There were four lecturers/professors with less than forty students. We assigned each other classes to teach, preparing the lectures and working with the students. It included the practical application of the practical courses. I taught Systematic Theology courses, Hermeneutics, Pastoral Epistles, Homiletics, Evangelism, Pastoral Counseling, Paul's Epistles, Church Administration, Church History, etc. For the practical application of evangelism, I used to organize evangelism outreach in the local villages.

The students would walk more than fifty kilometers to the village of Vimba and invite people to come for the revival meetings, starting on Fridays, Saturdays and we would conclude on Sundays with a Sunday service many people gave their lives to Jesus, and we would welcome them. Those who gave their lives to Jesus Christ would bring their charms, talismans, ritual artifacts, sacred clothes, and so on. The students were on fire for the Lord. The same strategy

I used for evangelism outreach when I was a Pastor in Mutare District, is the same strategy I used with the students at RBC. The time I spent at Rusitu Bible College as a Lecturer/Professor was valuable as I imparted knowledge, and Christian and moral values to students as we prepared them to be Ministers, missionaries, and into the world-wide missions.

When we moved from Zimbabwe to the USA in 2008, I had completed my Bachelor of Divinity/M. Div. degree from Africa University and master's in educational education policy studies and planning from Zimbabwe Open University. I was admitted to Puritan Reformed Theological Seminary in Grand Rapids for my second master's but now in Theology and graduated in May 2010. After completing my master's degree, I was admitted the same year to study for my Doctorate at Southern Baptist Theological Seminary and graduated in 2016. I was then hired by the North American Mission Board as a missionary/church planter in Greater Seattle. We relocated from Louisville, Kentucky to Kent where we planted a church, Bread of Life International Fellowship in June 2016. In 2019, I was invited to join the Center for Theology and Missions faculty as a professor, in Seattle, Washington. I was assigned to teach Systematic Theology, Church Leadership/Administration, and Biblical Counseling, with three credits each course. The relational approach to education in which students and teachers are encouraged to relate at a deeper level, to develop and cultivate the relationship among professors with students in such a way as to bridge education and empathy with the students.

Chapter Five: A Clinical & Spiritual/Biblical Counselor

This chapter gives a glimpse of the Clinical Pastoral Education program and the expectations to fulfill the requirements of Clinical and Spiritual Care. I will introduce the chapter with the most fundamental nitty-gritty of the program by submitting my final evaluations of Levels I and II of the CPE. I have studied my five units at MultiCare Health Systems, two of which were at Good Samaritan Hospital and three as a resident at Tacoma General Hospital. The models used in this chapter are from "Advanced Holistic Healing," by Dr. Annette Gildemann.

I was motivated by the desire to fulfill the Great Commission (Matt. 28:18-20) to reach out to people who are hurting and to assist patients with spiritual care needs. I anticipate being a certified APEC educator. I joined the ministry of spiritual care to contribute and learn about how to evaluate and assess patients' spiritual needs and be able to discharge my duties as a spiritual care practitioner for the well-being of the patients. I desire to serve the patients who are in the hospital with dignity and respect and to give them spiritual care and support. I have a passion as well as compassion to serve the patients who are sick and are in despair because of their sicknesses, loss of their loved ones, and their family affairs. To minister to patients who need spiritual care and moral support motivates me.

Some of the central themes and core values of my faith are redemption by grace alone without works (Eph. 2:8-9), Soteriology, Christology, Pneumatology, Trinity, Eschatology, Parousia, Eternity, Sanctity of life, life after death with Christ. My core values are Biblical based on the conception of life as a zygote, fetus, infant, baby, to adulthood is regarded as precious life and as such must be respected and not be terminated in abortion. My core values also pattern to husband and wife i.e., male and female joined together in holy matrimony.

The Lord's Supper plays an important part in my pastoral functioning because it signifies Christ's body being broken and represented by the bread and the wine, representing his blood which was shed for our transgressions. It also signifies unity, fellowship, and communion as one body of believers, koinonia. Baptism also plays an important part in my pastoral functioning because it signifies the death and the resurrection of Christ.

The operation theology has developed this unit by giving me new insights about spiritual care and not focusing on myself or my agenda but instead focusing on the patient's spiritual and emotional needs. Chaplaincy is about focusing on the patient and his relatives and friends who are surrounding him/her. The operation theology has developed this unit by operating according to chaplaincy codes of conduct and following the patient-based spiritual needs, not the chaplain's desires or agenda. In that context, a spiritual care practitioner is open to meeting the needs of any patient who needs spiritual care without basing on religion, faith, or belief systems. My theology will not be affected by addressing patients' needs who have a different faith than mine.

My pastoral identity has been developed to be more embracive to other faiths and religions to discharge my duties as a spiritual caregiver practitioner. I have developed into being tolerant of other faiths, religions, and belief systems in or to a relevant, open-minded, and the best spiritual care practitioner.

Spiritual care is my passion, and my philosophy ministry is to be a servant leader, with humility, pursuing academic excellence, engaging with people of all different backgrounds, loving, and caring without employing transference and countertransference or using my academic profile but to meet patients at the point of their needs. The early years of my life shaped the philosophy of my ministry and enhanced by my academic and professional experience years later.

The major themes/relationships/events that impact my identity, affecting my functioning is the redemption in which Christ died for my sins and forgave my sins. Christ's resurrection means that I am also going rise again for eternity. My mind was transformed into the new man I am today and enhances my relationship with God, all humanity, and the universe. Christ's sacrifice on the cross compels me to sacrifice for other people in my community, with agape love. It also signifies unity, fellowship, and communion as one body of believers, koinonia.

They have impacted me positively in enhancing and strengthening my faith and belief in God as the sovereign Lord and it keeps me on track to please God. As a Pastor, I employ Pastoral care counseling to lead and guide the members of my church without any question. As a clinical and spiritual care professional, I give and guide them to find solutions to the problems and challenges they are facing in their lives, giving them a listening ear. You don't give or advise them on how to solve their challenges in life, but you allow them to solve their challenges by empowering them, exploring the possibilities, and facilitating and enabling them to their intended destinies and outcomes. In that context, my theology is challenged and my bias towards my pastoral duties is reversed. If a patient is healed, I cannot evaluate and assess the validity of the healing. With patients in the hospital, I am not attached to them, and I don't fully know or have intimate relationships with them. They are not mine but for the hospital and I leave them at the hospital while my church members I have them always and I have an intimate relationship with them.

The new insight or self-knowledge is a chaplain is a spiritual care practitioner for every patient regardless of their religion or faith. You do not have a right to preach or to convert/proselyte a patient to believe in your faith nor to ask him/her to invite Christ in his/her life. The CPE has changed my view of chaplaincy, a huge paradigm of thinking, perception, and understanding of a patient's worldview.

I always accept criticisms from my class peers and supervisor because they make me stronger and give me insights to check on my blind spots. I am glad that I can accept criticism without being upset or angry. It allows me to assess and assimilate the criticism without being confrontational. If the criticisms are genuine, honest, constructive, academic, and not personal, I accept criticisms. I received critiques with honor although I had to answer questions that were not clear.

The pieces of critique that touched me most were those which were affirming my compassion, my gifts, loving people, and caring for them. Those critiques encouraged me and uplifted my soul. However, some criticisms stirred my heart and challenged me about the verbatims that I presented that missed a lot of important things. Some of the verbatims are those that were done, probably influenced by my theological belief systems and my conclusion and according to my faith. I was touched by two of my verbatims, one about suicide and abortion which were very spoken of and brought to my blind spots.

My espoused theology takes the Bible literally and applies it to one's life in the practical sense. It teaches that every prayer should end with "In Jesus's Name" and with an "Amen." It also teaches that if someone is not a Christian, you must share with him/her about Jesus and invite him/her to receive Christ as Lord and Savior. It teaches that the Bible is the only Holy Bible, not any other book. It teaches that Jesus Christ is the way, the truth, and the life and that no one comes to the Father, God except through Jesus alone. The operation theology at Good Samaritan Hospital teaches the opposite of espoused theology. It teaches that if someone is not a Christian as I am, the chaplain does not pray in the name of Jesus and should not say "Amen." It teaches that you are not a pastor in the hospital but a chaplain.

My theological meaning of CPE experience is that the theology of CPE is different in the fact that theology is the study of God. CPE does not necessarily talk about God in the sense of God of the universe, but it is relative to the contextualized gods or spirituality of different patients according to their belief systems or faiths. I used to relate theology to monotheistic beliefs or faiths but now I presume that in CPE, theology means the study of deity in a relative sense, according to the patient's deity. Patients have different belief systems, religions, and faiths. As such, the chaplain must understand each patient's beliefs and faith and explore with him/her how they connect with their deity.

To know the patient's faith or religion and explore with him/her his/her religion and to understand how they connect with their deity. Not to act like a pastor or a counselor but as a chaplain. To work as a team with doctors, nurses, therapists, and all social workers. Act promptly and timely when you receive a Telmediq when you are on-call. To receive criticism with a cheerful outlook without taking it personally from your peers and supervisor. Accept corrections from your supervisor, class peers, and preceptors. To write chat notes with clarity and not to express the emotions of the patient except if they come from the patient, directly. To be able to write verbatim that focuses on the patient without pushing him/her into your agenda or what you desire. It should be patient-driven. To dress in casual business attire, to be clean always from the head, mouth, and up to the toes. To respect all the patients, the supervisor, class peers, and their views and beliefs. To love unity in diversity and tolerate other cultures and racial differences. To critique class peers fairly and justly without any bias.

Brett, you are a pleasant man. You are honest in your criticisms of your peers. I love Augustine's approach and how he, analyzes issues. The strengths of Augustine are that you are bold to explore the needs of the patient regardless of his/her situation without any bias towards the patient. Augustine's race, ascent, and culture should not hinder your growth. You are a full package as a chaplain and your passion for the patients' welfare will make you an even stronger and vibrant chaplain. Augustine, you were trying to teach the group to be bold and honest and to uphold the chaplaincy code of conduct to the highest standard. My relationship with Augustine is very warm and we share the same challenges of our ascents, backgrounds, and ministry from Africa. We love each other as brothers. It is a great privilege to know you, Augustine. Your feedback was right on the spot. You are smart, honest, and bold. You are going to be a great chaplain and father. Keep on doing what is important to build up people. Your sense of humor, and laughter, makes me realize that we were meant to be brothers forever.

Alick, you are a strong and enthusiastic man with a bold heart to explore things without fear. You are strong-willed, and you have a great passion for exploring issues with the patients to get impedimental solutions to their challenges. Your boldness and fearless character might have developed more because you are a chaplain in the Navy. Your strength is that you have a strong passion for doing good for those who are in dilemma, and you want to offer help as a chaplain. You are a family person who loves finance, dearly. Crossing your culture to marry someone who is not your race tells a lot about your character without biases. Your experience as a pastor and chaplain in the Navy has earned your intellectual prowess to be able to discern and discharge your duties fairly. Reggie, you need to improve not to try to make decisions for the patients as a counselor, but you must adjust to chaplaincy codes, not to be a pastor or a counselor. Your compassionate heart compels you to offer some help to the patients as a chaplain. You have an exciting potential to be one of the best chaplains. Reggie tries to teach the group to combine compassion with professionalism in chaplaincy. I enjoyed your honest feedback, which was well organized. Your easy forgiving spirit is God and I admire your intellectual capacity.

Grace you are a loving woman, soft-spoken and with a quiet character but with a very powerful intellectual ability to discern, articulate, and analyze people, issues, situations, and circumstances and come to an informed conclusion. You are smart, initiative-taking, and diligent. Your strength is in your ability to probe and explore with the patients to understand the patient's social and spiritual needs. Your compassion and care for the patient earns your trust in the patient. Alicia, you can empathize with the patient to the extent that you can take on extra tasks that are not in your job description to make the patient feel loved and cared for. Alicia, you can become a great chaplain if you become more open and friendly with your peers and anyone who wants to know you better. But your pleasant character diffuses any weaknesses that can become your strengths. You tried to teach the group to be more strategic in performing our clinical duties and presenting their verbatims. You are kind and generous and you want to help anyone who is in need. Your soft and calm character has tremendous potential to make you one of the best chaplains on the block!

I have learned to be content with all the critiques that I received from all my peers and my supervisor. I have learned to focus on the patient instead of coming up with my agenda and pushing my belief systems or faith to the patients. Instead, I can explore issues with them their belief systems, faith, moral and social orientations. I must be open, caring, compassionate, and willing to accept my peers in their kinds of beliefs and faiths. I have learned that I am an enthusiastic chaplain and pastor. I have learned that I make many mistakes, and have many blind spots, and realize that I give apologies and apologies in many instances, even if it is not necessary. All my peers are loving and caring and yet they were able to give constructive criticism without any bias at all. They were able to adjust to a caring mode after debates, opposed opinions, about their convictions. It is a formidable group of people who want to excel in their chaplaincy profession. I love them all and I am so grateful to learn with them.

Jenny, you are one of the greatest scholars and enthusiastic supervisors I have ever met. My experience with you has been warm, loving, caring, and yet with academic excellence and intellectually solid. You guided me very well with my peers in my clinical and class times. You gave me great advice about my peers, patients, and staff team. You are very smart, enthusiastic, and have academic prowess. Jenny's strengths are observed as she integrates academic expertise with spiritual repertoire and advises students not to be pastors nor counselors in the hospitals but to be devoted chaplains who discharge their professional duties with a sense of responsibility, excellence, accountability, and ownership. Jenny, your edges are that you become more system-oriented but at the same time, you balance it with humor, jokes, and open laughter that diffuses any of your weaknesses. You are a great supervisor, and I am so grateful to have Jenny as my supervisor. Jenny, you are kind and compassionate and you act quickly when asked a question or to address a need. You are always there to assist interns. The book reviews you gave us to review were educational and helpful, especially "The Lost Art of Listening," by Michael P. Nichols.

Jenny you were trying to teach the group to let each student grow and develop his/her potential to be vibrant, enthusiastic, and spiritual caregivers without compromising their belief systems, faith, and convictions in the process and those of the patients. Jenny, you taught the class to be able to develop listening skills and explore their patients' anxieties, worries, and concerns without pushing their agendas, belief systems, faith, convictions, and social and moral orientations. You taught us to love, care for, and support each other. We are all grateful for Jenny's skills, passion, love, care, and support that she gives to each student to succeed in chaplaincy.

CPE is a great program that teaches chaplain-interns some skills, proactiveness, empathy, patience, accountability, and professionalism. The changes that I can suggest about the CPE program are about the clinical hours that are required to be completed. The 300 hours of clinical time and 100 hours for the class are huge for a full-time employee anywhere. These are too many hours that are required for one unit. If four units are required for one to be recognized as a full-time chaplain, and yet four hundred hours are required for just one unit, that makes it a full-time job already. Some of the people who have full-time jobs yet like the training will find it difficult to do this training. However, CPE has given me some skills to use both in the hospitals and the church, counseling as well as my family. It has given me opportunities to deal with my biases, emotions, and challenges, and to see the scope of chaplaincy. Clinical Pastoral Education title does not match with the pastoral education. Chaplaincy and pastoral duties and expectations are two different animals, why then is it called "pastoral" when pastoral skills are not allowed in chaplaincy? The contrast is vast. I will propose to drop the word "pastoral" and replace it with "Spiritual Care Professional/Practitioner".

The group is very diverse which includes Africans, Asians, and Americans. It is a blended group so beautifully, with different backgrounds, convictions, and social experiences. The students' characters and religious affiliations were so much represented to bring great flavor to the table to discuss, debate, and differ in opinions and belief systems. The life ministry peer process group allowed students to be vulnerable in the skits of a chaplain and a patient, challenging their comfort zones. I enjoyed thoroughly the dynamics of the live ministry process group that unfolded in this unit.

The meaningful concepts that I took away are reflective listening to patients, exploring with them their emotional and spiritual needs, understanding the concepts of the patient-chaplain relationship, and teamwork with the hospital staff. Some of the meaningful concepts taken away from CPE are pastoral formation, competence, and reflection, theological evaluation and reflection, and evaluation in general. I have applied some of these concepts in my pastoral ministry to counsel, teach, and use them with my staff for evaluating performance using the 'smart' goals in my church and community. I have also used these concepts in counseling and teaching.

My relationship with people of other faiths has been good but not the best. It is always a great challenge to get out of one's comfort zone. However, I was able to learn their faith and belief systems. I was able to explore with them their spiritual care needs in their faiths and understood how they connect with their deity and then come to their conclusions according to their faiths.

My interaction with the patients was one of the most fulfilling of my clinical training. I was able to hear what was in their hearts, looked them in their eyes, eyeballs to eyeballs, heard their breathing and groaning in pain, held their warm and cold hands, prayed with them, heard their spirits departing from their motionless bodies as the doctors stretched the curtains behind them as their lives ended. It was a time of personal introspection of life and death, I placed myself into their shoes and imagined how my wife, my mother, my children, and all my consanguinity would feel when I gasped for my last breath as my soul departed from my mortal body into eternity with my Lord, Christ Jesus, and joining other saints. It was a sobering experience but also with great joy to serve them.

I have encountered and interacted with great nurses in my clinical training at Good Samaritan Hospital. However, some were not that friendly, not warm too, and gave me the cold shoulder. People are not all the same. Some are kind and some are not, but I managed to treat everyone equally with high respect, dignity, and honor regardless of their attitudes and temperaments. I collaborated well with social workers and other staff who were helpful, resourceful, and of great encouragement. The volunteers also did a superb job!

This CPE unit was challenging for me at the beginning as I am also a Ph.D. candidate, majoring in Medical Anthropology at the University of Washington, Seattle main campus, a minister at a local church, and a father of five children with my wife. I had to suspend my semesters at the university to concentrate and to give all my time to this CPE unit. I was able to do my clinical 300+ hours as a volunteer at Good Samaritan Hospital as well as write and present five verbatims, chat notes at the hospital, visit patients, do on-call duties, and both midterm and final evaluations. I was able to interact with my peers very well as well as my supervisor. I was willing to be vulnerable, to be critiqued, and evaluated based on my academic experience, and spirituality, and to discharge chaplain duties.

I can introspect myself and be able to reflect on the things I have done and come to my conclusions with resolutions to change and improve. In other words, I am very cautious of what I do. If I miss the opportunity to see my mistakes but when friends highlight my blind spots, I can reflect on the issues and analyze my mistakes, and then I can accept my mistakes, apologize, and move forward. I try to be humble and diligent in dealing with my shortcomings. Evaluation of my actions, my speech, my comments, and my shortcomings gives me the strength to improve to be a better person and professional chaplain.

GOAL 1: Pastoral Formation

- *My goal*: My goal is to maintain boundaries while offering pastoral care.
- *Indication*: I know I love people and I do not intend to build a long and mutual relationship with patients but to be professional. Sometimes I do build long-term relationships with people, and I enjoy these relationships. This can sometimes make my visits more of a social visit rather than a chaplaincy visit. Something I would like to pay attention to

- *Methods and resources*: I hope to use verbatim seminars, and feedback from my peers and my supervisor, and also be willing to learn from my blind spots.
- *The ways I may sabotage myself*: I might discharge my best spiritual care to patients but at the same time, develop relationships with the patients which is not professionalism.

  Achievement: I was able to be professional in giving spiritual care to the patients instead of trying to develop or build relationships, then I now know that I have achieved my goal.

GOAL 2. Pastoral Competence

- *My goal*: I want to learn to give critique fairly and honestly.
- *Indications:* I know I don't like giving critiques and will usually just compliment people for what they are not.
- *Methods and resources*: I hope to use verbatim seminars, and process group times to offer critique to my peers and supervisor.
- *The ways I may sabotage myself*: I might give a very soft critique or just say the same things someone has just said.
- *Achievement*: I have offered clear and constructive critiques to each one of my peers and my supervisor. I have achieved my goals.

GOAL 3. Pastoral Reflection
- *My goal*: To be able to listen and let the patient talk about their emotions and spiritual needs.
- *Indications*: I know I have vast theological education and pastoral experience hence I know how to display pastoral care

that can hinder the true needs of the patient. That might hinder patients from their cocoons of spiritual and emotional needs.

- *Methods and resources*: I hope to use my peers' feedback verbatim, group process times, and my supervisor's critique and advice.
- *The ways I may sabotage myself*: By allowing my theological education and pastoral experience to run the show.

Achievement: My goal has been achieved and I have realized that the center of spiritual care is on the patient. I have made space for the patient to talk, facilitating conversation, and I have not let my education and knowledge run the show.

My first goal was to maintain boundaries while offering pastoral care: I believe I have achieved this goal as I was able to maintain boundaries as I offered pastoral and spiritual care to the patients. I was very much aware to keep away from pastoring or counseling the patients but instead, I was only offering them spiritual care as well as exploring with them their spiritual belief systems and faiths. They would come to their solutions according to their beliefs and faith. I am now able to maintain those boundaries without confusing them.

My second goal was to learn to give critiques fairly and honestly: I have achieved my goal of being able to give my peers fair and honest critiques. It was hard at first to give honest critiques because of fear of not hurting my peers' feelings but with friendship and good rapport with each of them, I was able to be honest with my evaluation and assessment of any verbatim presented and be able to critique it fairly. My goal was achieved.

My third goal was to be able to listen and let the patient talk about their emotions and spiritual needs: I achieved this goal as I allowed the patients to talk about their emotions while I was listening. Listening is an art, and it is required as it is one of the skills of a chaplain that needs to be learned. The book, "The Lost Art of Listening" by Michael P. Nichols is a powerful book that has taught me to realize that I needed to listen more to the patient's needs. If one is not a good listener, ultimately one becomes a bad chaplain. The focus should be on the patient not for the chaplain to bring his/her agenda, theology, counseling, or to give advice. Listening is the opposite of doing things for a patient. I achieved my goal of being able to listen and understand the needs of the patient. I have grown in understanding the importance of listening as art for CPE's thrust.

My strengths are that I am compassionate, able to listen to the patient's emotional and spiritual needs and loving and caring for the patients. I can accept criticism easily, I don't hold grudges, I can forgive easily, and I can relate with anyone without any bias. I treat people equally regardless of their race or ethnicity. I have leadership skills because of my experience and academic achievements. I have three Masters' degrees and one of them is in Biblical Counseling which helps me in counseling outside the hospital. I have a Doctorate in Educational Leadership and I am currently studying for my second Doctorate (Ph.D.) in Medical Anthropology at the University of Washington. Academically, I am strong. I have written seven books available on Amazon.com, Barnes and Noble bookstores, and other retail channels. My support base is my family who are loving and caring, my wife and five children. I can work with anyone or any institution without any problem. I can communicate and interact with any patient to meet their spiritual care and needs. As a chaplain, I don't bring with me my academic achievement and Pastoral experience.

My growing edge is that I do not fully understand the cultures of various people in America. They are diverse people in America and their cultures are different. Sometimes I find it very difficult to resonate with some patients, especially when they hear my accent. They switch and start to question me where I come from and how and when I came to America. I have learned the skills, however, from this unit to divert their questions instead, to zero in on themselves not myself because the visit should focus on themselves, not myself. It is, indeed, a superb skill that I found is working well. Also, one of my growing edges is to bring in my theology, faith, counseling skills, and belief systems to the patient while I am talking to them. I have learned, however, from this unit that I should not bring my baggage with me when I am talking to the patients. I must listen to them. My growing edges have been dashed with some of the skills offered in this unit, thank God! I sometimes apply my experience and education when talking to patients, especially those who question my educational qualifications and my experience. Some of them would say when I entered their rooms, "Are you a doctor?" and my response would be, "Yes, I am a spiritual Doctor, or the physician of the soul, or the chaplain!" This will usually be a humorous response just to dispel any suspicion or tension with some patients. It will be a good introduction to engage with the patients to start a conversation. I did not do it to all the patients but only some of them.

"Then he came to Bethsaida, and they brought a blind man to him and begged him to touch him. So, he took the blind man by the hand and led him outside of the town. When he had spit on his eyes and put his hands on him, Jesus asked, "Do you see anything?" He looked up and said, "I see people; they look like trees, walking around." Once again Jesus puts his hands on the man's eyes. Then his eyes were opened, his sight was restored, and he saw everything clearly," (Mark 8:22-23).

Before I started CPE, this unit, I saw people as living beings but now I see them as living souls who need spiritual care. I was blind but now I see, I can listen and understand and empathize with them. I can be in the pit with them (Psalm 22) and walk out of the pit with them (Psalm 23). I no longer see people as trees, walking around but I see people as people. Christ has opened my blind eyes. That's what this unit has done for me! I am so thankful for our supervisor, Luz, my incredible peers, staff chaplains in Good Samaritan Hospital, Richard, and Nicole, for their moral and physical support, and of course, Annette, who found us a wonderful supervisor amid crisis to find one. I am so thankful to God, Almighty, for giving me good health during this unit and my family, of course, who was always with me even if I was not always there for them.

VERBATIM I EXAMPLE

Verbatims are interactions between the CPE student with the patients in the hospital setting and then the written verbatims are then brought to the class to be critiqued, assessed, and evaluated, and the feedback is given to the student who would have presented by the peers and certified educator. These platforms are designed to help the students improve their skills to identify the emotions, feelings, and needs of the patients or staff and be able to apply the learned interventions. The following are some of the examples of verbatims I presented to the class.

Title of this Verbatim: "Deciding end of Life."

I.   DATA ABOUT CPE STUDENT AND PATIENT

CPE Student:
My name is Sam S. Mhlanga, and I am originally from Zimbabwe in Southern Africa. My denomination is the Southern Baptist Convention. I am an African in my fifties and I am married to Judith, and we have five children.

Patient's name:
James is 65 years old, and he is a male Caucasian. He is not married, and he lives with his sister, Grace. He is a devoted Christian, Lutheran.

Date Visited patient/family:
Length of Visit: 50 minutes

Staff Consultations: Before I saw the patient, I checked with the nurse who told me about the patient's condition and how he was processing his diagnosis, wanting to end his life. When I entered James's room, I was aware of what he wanted to do, and he had asked for a chaplain to confirm his decision. He was so emotional about his decision. The nurse had debriefed me about the patient's condition and what he wanted.

Medical Diagnosis: Colon cancer and he had lost hearing in both ears. You had to shout louder for him to hear. He had benign prostate, chronic hip pain, duodenal ulcer, sinus headache, acute respiratory failure with hypoxia, and skin onychomycosis. He was in palliative care on the 8th floor.

Reason for presenting this visit: I am bringing this verbatim to get some insights as to what to process with the patient when he tells you that he wants to end his life, according to his faith but contrary to his faith.

My three goals:

1. **My first goal is to understand my feelings and those of patients.**

I will continue to have this goal with the purpose of improving my understanding of my emotions and those of patients. I plan to fulfill this goal by listening with my heart to patients' emotions.

2. **My second goal is to reflect on patients' feelings and not to question them.**

I will fulfill this goal by intentionally, putting on the mindset, repeating it in my mind when I enter patients' rooms, "Reflection, Reflection, Reflection", "Not being inquisitive."

3. **My third goal is to be open and willing to learn and reflect on patients' stories and their past experiences.**

I intend to fulfill this goal by intentionally, thick-listening patients' stories and their past experiences, showing them with facial expressions and nodding to encourage and to show them that I am interested in their stories.

II. OBSERVATION AND AWARENESS

A. <u>First impressions and observations:</u> The door was open, and the patient was lying on the bed and the room was full of medical staff doing different things on James. James was speaking very loudly it was because he had lost hearing in both ears. I finally had an opportunity too to visit with him, late in the after trying several times to see him. His sister, Grace, was with him interpreting for him because James did not understand what people were saying clearly. His sister was attending to him to make sure that he was feeling comfortable. I liked the way James's sister was so close to him and gave him what he needed.

B. <u>EQ - Awareness of self before the visit:</u> I was aware of my emotions and feelings after reading James's diagnosis. It was an Epic order on the 8th floor, which is not my floor, but the preceptor asked me to go and visit the patient, on his floor, a palliative unit.

III. SPIRITUAL CARE ENCOUNTER WITH THE LIVING HUMAN DOCUMENT:

Please identify the speakers; for example: C=Chaplain, P=Patient, S=Sister

speaker	Dialogue, spoken and non-verbal	Internal experience – feelings/thoughts/self-awareness
C1	*(The door was opened but the curtain was pulled in)* Knock,	*I was checking to see if he was James and if he would*

	knock. May I come in? My name is Chaplain Sam, one of the Chaplains at Tacoma Hospital. Are you James? It is right now. It will take taking 20 minutes or so depending on our conversation.	*allow me into his room. I was adhering to AIDET, Acknowledge, Introduce, Duration, Explanation, and Thank You.*
P1	Yes. I am James. Who are you? (*Whizzing as he was gasping for more oxygen*)	*He asked me if I could come closer to him as he could not hear me.*
C2	Sure, let me come closer to you. How are you doing, James today? (He *seemed to be in agony*).	*I could imagine the pain James was going through with colon cancer, benign prostate, chronic hip pain, duodenal ulcer, sinus headache, acute respiratory failure with hypoxia, and skin onychomycosis.*
P2	Thank you, Chaplain Sam, for coming. I want to ask you a question. You are a Chaplain, are you a Christian?	*I had to be honest with James that I was a Christian.*
C3	Yes, I am a Christian. How are you doing today, you may ask your question, James.	*I knew that James was a Christian in his profile.*
S1	Chaplain Sam says he is a Christian. You wanted to ask a Chaplain. He is here now. You can ask him. (*James's sister,*	*I felt empathy for James. I had compassion and sympathy for James. It reminded me of my*

	Grace said it in a loud voice in his ears, closer to him).	*grandmother. We used to speak to her loudly in her ears because she could not hear clearly.*
C4	Yes, I am here. Do you want to ask me a question? Go ahead, James, I am listening.	
P4	Yes, I am a Christian Chaplain Sam. I have lived a quality life. I am 65 years old now. All the diseases that I have are causing my health to decline. I don't expect to have a quality life again.	*I was eager to hear his question and I was feeling empathetic for James because his body was shutting down, you could tell.*
C5	I am listening to James. It sounds like you have an important question to ask.	*I was trying to affirm what he was saying.*
P5	As a Christian, will God accept me in heaven if I pull the plug off voluntarily? I know that I will not have any quality life anymore because God gave me a quality life already.	*I was silent, listening with my heart.*
S2	My brother has been asking this question for some time now. He is saying he wants to die now because his body is tormenting him day and night. He has been	*I thought of this tricky question. I began to reflect on one of my goals to reflect, reflect, and reflect. I am not to ask questions*

	saying he wants to die because he does not see the reason to live a substandard and he knows he not recover. May you please speak to him about God. He wants assurance that God will accept him in heaven if he tells the doctors to remove the machines.	*and I do not teach or give him my answers.*
P6	Yes, Chaplain Sam, may you please confirm to me that God will accept me. That he will not punish me for allowing my body to succumb to my illness, voluntarily because I do not want to live anymore. God gave me a quality life.	*As he was talking, I was thick listening, trying to understand his emotions, to connect with him in his pain.*
C7	I hear you, James. It sounds like you have difficulty deciding your life	*I was thinking that I could tell him what God says about murder and about the destiny of the murderers in the Bible in which he believes. I refused in my mind to allow myself to be dragged into that discussion.*
P7	Chaplain Sam, please confirm that I will be ok with God. I know I am a born-again Christian and I know that when	*I was struggling to block all the teaching and advising mentality that was pushing me through*

	I die, I will go to heaven because I received Christ in my life my salvation is secure.	*my mind. I told myself, the professor should sit down on the chair and shut up.*
C8	It sounds like you have a good connection with your God. It sounds like you have a good understanding of your belief system and your faith's teachings.	*I was empathic to James' health challenges and the decisions that he must make. I told myself that I was not a part of his decision.*
P8	Chaplain Sam, why not be able to help me with my decision? I am frustrated.	*I suppressed my teaching mode.*
C9	The decision is all up to you, James. I understand what you are going through. The decision rests with you and your family.	*I was coming alongside and listening to James with my heart as he narrated his ordeal.*

| S3 | Chaplain Sam, James wanted you to confirm that if he allows the machines to be removed and he dies, God will not hold him accountable. | *Silence, and thick listening.* |
| C10 | About pulling the plug, it is on James and the family. I cannot make any decision for James. | *I reflected on his strong emotions and feelings about the final decision he was to make. What I said in my mind about Christian faith, was that his salvation is secure in* |

		Christ no matter how one does with his life. The result is that Christians' salvation is secure., they cannot lose salvation even if they commit suicide. However, even if I knew, I chose not to tell him but allowed him to make his final decision.
P10	I know your answer Chaplain Sam because we both believe in God, including my sister, Grace. Thank you for listening and presenting me. If I don't see here on earth, I will see in heaven, brother.	*I was feeling compassionate and empathetic to James and his sister, Grace, as they had to figure out the final decision.*
C11	Thank you, James, for allowing me to hear about your health challenges and for allowing me to listen and get to know your sister, Grace. Hope you make the best decision for yourself and your family. Is there anything I can do before I leave?	*I came closer to James and wished him the best in making the final decision.*
P11	Yes, Chaplain Sam. Please, I need a prayer. May you please, pray that God will help me to make my final decision so that	*I stood there, thick-listening, compassionate, understanding my feelings too.*

	God will be happy with me and let me into heaven.	
C12	Yes, we may pray. We held hands, hands, three of us.	*We were like a family, and I prayed for James, knowing in my heart that whatever decision he made, it would be the best decision for their family and that God would see him through*
P12	*I am at peace now with God even if you did not tell me. The fact that you are here gives me peace.*	*Silence and deep listening.*
C13	Let's pray. *"Our gracious Heavenly God, I pray for James to hear him as he asks you to give him direction as to what to do with his life. May you to what to do. Thank you to his sister, Grace who is beside him, supporting him all the way. Give strength and peace as she comes alongside her dear brother James. them comfort and peace. Amen.*	*I felt the presence of God.*

P14	Thank you, Chaplain Sam, I am so grateful for your service and your support.	*I could feel the cold hands of James.*

C14	You are welcome. Thank you for allowing the space to be with you.	.
P15	All the blessings to you!	

C15	Thank you! (*Then I left the room*)	

Gildemann asserts, "It is important to state that the focus of the chaplain documentation is on the spiritual, relational, and emotional aspects of the person and should rarely include biomedical information… Documenting serves to help the patient to be seen in their human fullness."[18] Gildemann highlights the fundamental facets of Clinical and Spiritual Care to patients and their family and friends. She continues, "To move toward clarity in the documentation the RAIN format is integrated into the HARP-M spiritual assessment model. RAIN stands for Reason for Visit, Assessment, Intervention, and Next Steps."[19]

Reason for Visit: Met with patient per Epic order.

Assessment: **of** **spiritual** **needs/resources:** Patient communicated spiritual distress related to peace.

[18] Gildemann, Annette, Advanced Holistic Healing, (Booknook.biz Publishers, 2020), 72.
[19] Ibid. 73.

Needs:

The patient said he feels he has lived a quality life and does not want to continue to live a sub-standard life with his illness. He reported that he had decided to be put in MCO, voluntarily. James said he wanted to confirm if he had made the right decision to be extubated, by choice. James said that he wrestles with his personal decision and finds peace about that decision. He asked for a prayer to be able to make his final decision about the end of his life plan. His sister, Grace was on his besides, comforting and supporting him.

Strengths:

James engaged in self-reflection, and reporters can ask for help and are willing to accept it when offered. The patient shared a connection with God that supports their ability to cope. The patient described their family as very caring and supportive which the patient says helps them to have hope, especially his sister, Grace. James reported that he has regular practices, including prayer that give hope.

Intervention:

- Explored sources of peace/comfort to help find peace.

- Identified relationship strengths to equip the patient for positive coping.

- Used the patient's faith tradition (Christian) to ease spiritual distress.

- Provided prayer to provide solidarity in grief/comfort to support the patient.

Next Steps/Follow-up: Spiritual needs addressed, consult complete. The spiritual care team remains available for additional support as needed.

Dr. Rev. Sam S. Mhlanga: (Chaplain Resident). D.Ed., M.Ed., M.Th., M.Div., PhD (cand).

Spiritual Care Team remains available for additional support as needed:

VI.   REFLECTION ON THE VISIT

1.   EQ, emotional self-awareness
   - I felt sad to see James in such a condition when I heard his whizzing, gasping for more oxygen, and multiple diagnoses. I entered deep grief for James and her sister Grace who has been with him. Grace demonstrated what a family should be with love and care for her sibling. I was now aware of what James was going through and the difficult decision he was to make.

   - EQ, awareness of others' emotions
   - I was aware of the emotions of James in making a final decision about his life to end it.

2.   At which points did you feel connected/disconnected?
- I felt connected with James as a Christian.

- I felt disconnected from James when he insisted that I should confirm his decision to end his life because I don't believe in euthanasia.

a.   What strategy of disconnection did you use?

3.   What were your strengths?
My strengths were action, reflection, and action with James about her multiple diagnoses coming alongside her in her sickness and empathizing with her.

4.   What did you struggle with?
I struggled to avoid advising and teaching.

5.   State what you would do differently during the visit by listing specifically in the dialogue where and what you might have done. As you look at alternative relational stances, do you have any insights about what caused you to take a particular stance, and why now would you choose something different?
- I would do differently by listening and reflecting on James's emotions and feelings, deeply without too much probing.

6.   What factors in your personal history, culture, or family system may have influenced your assessment and response to this situation? Did the encounter remind you of anyone/ any situation in your life? How might this have impacted on the visit?

- I come from Zimbabwe and my personal history, culture, family systems, and faith background have influenced me in my assessments and response to situations. However, having lived in America for 15 years I now lean to American culture on my assessment.

Spiritual Assessment of patient/family: (the sentence from your chart notes)

1. Based on your assessment what did you do? (Intervention – describe what you did in the encounter)

Intervention:

- Explored sources of peace/comfort to help find peace.
- Identified relationship strengths to equip the patient for positive coping.
- Used the patient's faith tradition (Christian) to ease spiritual distress.
- Provided prayer to provide solidarity in grief/comfort to support patients.

2. What did you learn about your pastoral role and function?

- I learned that deep listening, coming alongside the patients in their difficult situations, and understanding my personal feelings and those of my patients are the foundation of pastoral role and function. I have learned to embrace every religion of my patients without any biases.

3.   What learning goals did you work on during this visit? I believe I worked on three of my goals in this visit.

- My first goal is to understand my emotions and those of patients.
- My second goal is to reflect on patients' feelings and not to question them.
- My third goal is to be open and willing to learn and reflect on patients' stories and their past experiences.

4.   What Level I/II outcomes did you work on?

- Level II

5.   Describe the learning needs you identified from this visit.
- I need to listen more, understand my emotions and those of my patients more, and come alongside them in an empathetic way. Not to ask questions but to listen and reflect on the patient's emotions.

6.   Theological Reflection
What sacred or archetypal story or image comes up for you as you reflect on this visit?

- The image that comes up in my mind is Job who was so sick to the extent of death, but he did not curse or blame God regardless of his illness.

7.	Write a prayer or mindful or heartfelt thoughts for your patient and another for yourself.

Lord, may you guide James and Grace, his sister in peace, strength, and comfort to manage, and give James's guidance as he makes his final decision about his wife. Please, Lord, give them your Spirit and peace, to endure this difficult time. Amen.

VERBATIMS II EXAMPLE

Title of this Verbatim: "Multiple Grief"

**I.	DATA ABOUT CPE STUDENT AND PATIENT**

CPE Student:
My name is Sam S. Mhlanga.

Patient's name:
Natasha is 60 years old, and she is a female African American. She is divorced and she has 8 children and 18 grandchildren. She is a Christian, Pentecostal.

Date Visited patient/family:
Length of Visit: 45 minutes

Staff Consultations: Before I entered the room with the patient, I checked with the nurse who told me that the patient had COVID-19 positive and advised me to put on a gown, gloves, and glass shields. The nurse informed me that the patient needed spiritual and emotional support as she was grieving multiple deaths in her family.

When I entered Natasha's room, I was aware that she needed grief support and consolation. The nurse had debriefed me about the patient's condition and what she wanted from Spiritual Care.

Medical Diagnosis: CHF Exacerbation, ESRD Pneumonia/Covid-19 Positive. She was on the 6th floor, room 6---. Natasha was not showing any signs of illness, but she concentrated on the loss and grief of her loved ones.

Reason for presenting this visit: I am bringing this verbatim to demonstrate how the chaplain can come alongside a patient who has had multiple deaths in the family and also to get some insights as to how to process the grief of a patient who has been impacted with multiple deaths in the family.

My three goals:

1. My first goal is to name my emotions and those of patients.

2. My second goal is to reflect on patients' feelings and to ask generative questions, open-ended questions.

3. My third goal is to be open and willing to learn and reflect on patients' stories and their past experiences.

II.   OBSERVATION AND AWARENESS

C.   First impressions and observations: The door was closed; the patient was lying on the bed and the room was dark with dimmed lights. The patient's table was filled with empty plates showing that she had her lunch. I was impressed by the cleanliness of her room with some flowers on the window, with some dolls. Natasha had two phones on her bed and an iPad.

D. Awareness of self before the visit: I was aware of my emotions and feelings after reading the chart notes of a social worker and doctor. It was an Epic order on the 4th floor. This is not my floor but Jim's floor. He asked me to go and see the patient. First, I was worried why Jim had asked me to go to see the patient, and the patient was Covid-19 positive. In obedience, I went.

III. SPIRITUAL CARE ENCOUNTER WITH THE LIVING HUMAN DOCUMENT:

Please identify the speakers; for example: C=Chaplain, P=Patient, N=Nurse, Dr=Doctor, SW=Social Worker

speaker	Dialogue, spoken and non-verbal	Internal experience – feelings/thoughts/self-awareness
C1	*(The door was closed, and the room was dim)* Knock, knock. May I come in? My name is Chaplain Sam, one of the Chaplains at Tacoma Hospital. Are you Frank? Is it the right	*I was checking to see if he was Natasha and if she would allow me into her room. I was adhering to AIDET, Acknowledge, Introduce, Duration,*

	time now? I will take 20-30 minutes with you.	*Explanation, and Thank You.*
P1	Yes. I am Natasha. Who are you? Oh, you are a Chaplain. Yes, I called you because I am going through a lot. (*She asked me if I could take a chair and sit closer to her*).	*I thought that would be a long conversation and I got prepared to hear a lot from Natasha's heart.*
C2	yes, let me take the chair and come closer to you. Natasha, I hear you saying you are going through a lot. (*Her face looked worried and emotional*).	*I could imagine what she was going through with the multiple deaths in her family as the nurse debriefed me about Natasha's grief.*
P2	Thank you, Chaplain Sam, for coming. Yes, I am going through a terrible grief. My mother died four months ago. I am still grieving her, then my brother had a massive stroke and he died two weeks ago, followed by my aunt who collapsed and died a week ago. As if it was not enough, my daughter was found dead yesterday, and it is not known why and how she died. The Police are still investigating but they say they don't have evidence of the possible	*Natasha's family tragedy blew my mind. I could not comprehend the multiple deaths that her family was going through. I thought, where do I start? However, after settling my mind, composing myself, and deeply listening to Natasha, I thought this is the time to come alongside Natasha to fulfill one of my goals.*

	perpetrator (*Her eyes were tearing and emotional*).	
C3	I cannot imagine what you are going through, Natasha. It's one tragedy after another. First, your mother died four months ago, your brother had a stroke and died, your aunt collapsed and died, and your daughter was found dead, and the Police are still investigating who might have caused her death. Mm, it sounds like you are going through a lot, Natasha. I am very sorry to hear about such a painful and sad experience (*Her head was down and shaking her head*).	*I was reflecting and clarifying with Natasha to show that I was listening to her to her grieving stories and at the same time making sure that I was in line with her narration of the family tragedy.*
P3	Chaplain Sam, I called you because this is too much for me to bear alone in the Hospital. As we speak, they are burying my aunt who was close to me who was like my mother. I am here and I could not be at the funeral because I am here with covid. (*Natasha began to cry, bitterly*).	*I felt the sadness gripping me for Natasha and sad. I had compassion and sympathy for her. It reminded me of the tragedy when five family members perished in a car accident.*
C4	Oh, your aunt was like your mother, this sounds painful to lose your aunt. Your aunt meant	

	a lot to you. I can imagine, Natasha (*She was nodding her head*).	
P4	My brother had a massive stroke and he died two weeks ago. He left three children, but they are grown up. I was so close to my brother (*Looking up in the ceiling as if she was talking to God*).	*I thought, how do I comfort her and be alongside in a way that will make her cared for. I thought I was not inadequate.*
C5	I am so sorry Natasha for all the loss of your brother too. It started with your mother, then your brother and now your aunt. This should be very difficult to experience, Natasha (*Her eyes were tearing*).	*I was affirming her grieving, and I was so sad and frustrated as if I was the one.*
P5	As if it was not enough, Chaplain Sam, my daughter, was found dead in her apartment yesterday as I told you. It seems the spirit of death is following my family.	*I was silent, listening with my heart, and heartbroken at the same time. I resonated with Natasha when I connected with a tragedy that happened with our neighbors who perished in a car crash and five family members died on the spot.*

C6	I am so sorry for the loss of your daughter, Natasha. I hope the police will find the cause of her death and bring the perpetrator to justice if ever someone harmed her (*I saw her raising her hands up as I was speaking*).	*My heart was arching with sorry, and I was emotionally drained to hear tragedy after tragedy from Natasha.*
P6	I hope so but they say there is not enough evidence. However, I am suspicious of my cousin who lived with her. She said when she came back at night, she found her dead and naked. Can you imagine? She said that when she came to the apartment, she called the Police. But the doctors confirmed that she was dead between ten to twelve hours. God knows and if she played gimmicks with my daughter, God would judge her. (*She started crying, bitterly*).	*I could imagine her daughter lying in the room, dead. I was struggling to understand whether they were robbers who broke into the house, or if she might have committed suicide or if she overdosed. When that came to try to fathom what could have happened to her daughter.*
C7	Oh, the Police could not find enough evidence to implicate her on the death of your daughter.	*I was trying to come myself over all that I have heard so far. I remembered two of my goals, naming emotions of my patients and reflecting on them.*

P7	My family is haunted by the evil spirits who are trying to kill us all and I do not know how to stop it. I believe in God, and I am a Pentecostal, but I do not understand how God could allow this to happen to our family (*Shaking her head*).	*I was struggling to block all the preaching and advising mentality that was pushing me because in Africa, spiritualism is common, and I used to cast demons or evil spirits.*
C8	It sounds like you have a connection with God. In the past if there was death in your family, how did you process the death of your loved ones? Explore more about your understanding of evil spirits. (*I wanted to check how she relates with God and evil spirits*).	*I was checking if her spirituality helped her in the past. When she mentioned evil about the spirits, I resonated with that belief because the Bible talks about evil spirits that are against the children of God. In Africa, there are a lot of evil spirits in the villages.*
P8	I believe in Jesus Christ. God has been on my side, and I pray when I have such challenges like this. Chaplain Sam, as a Christian, in the past, our Pastor would come to pray and to comfort us with the word of God and pray with us. But the devil continues to fight against Christians as Paul talks about it in (Ephesians 6). (*Her eyes light*	*I thought if she believed in God, then at least she had faith to lean on. I thought to stop pursuing the topic of the evil spirits that she said may be attacking her family. However, it sounded like she believed that there may be some attack by the evil spirits and it's*

	up when she is talking about spiritual ware mentioned in Ephesians 6).	*important to her to pursue that worry.*
C9	It sounds like the evil spirits are real to you and you are worried about them attacking your family. Tell me more about them and prayer as you also mention prayer. It sounds like prayer means a lot to you in times like these. May you tell me more about what a prayer means to you.	*I was coming alongside and listening to Natasha as she continued to grieve as she narrated the ordeal was going through.*

	We defeat the evil spirits through prayer, but they keep on coming back to attack us as Christians. Prayer means a lot to me because prayer is how I communicate with God to ask, to thank Him, and to acknowledge Him as Lord, (*Natasha was not alive and actively involved in our conversation now. She had shifted from being sorrowful into fully engaged*).	*My heart was warmed to hear that Natasha has a source to get her strength during grieving.*
C10	I am glad to hear that you have the source of your strength.	*I reflected on her tragedy for a while in silence*

		understanding my emotions and feelings about her situation. I gave her a space to be silent and let her feel my presence.
P10	God has been my strength. Another thing I wanted to share with you is that one of my sons lives in New York. About a month ago, my son went to a bar with his cousins and friends. When they got to the bar, my son said he got sick with stomach pain. He returned to the hotel to sleep. He heard later that day that his cousins and friends had been shot and died. He said that a man came to the bar and started shooting everywhere. My son could have been shot but his life was spared because he got sick, and he had to return to the hotel room. God is always in the business of protecting my family but this time it is beyond my imagination (*Natasha went again into grief mode when she started talking about her son*	*I was baffled as I heard yet another story from Natasha.*

	who was spared because he went back to his hotel room, but his cousins and friends were shot in the bar).	
C11	I can imagine how now you feel Natasha with all that is going on with you and your family.	
P11	I have a lot to share Chaplain Sam, for you to come and listen to me. I am glad that you came and now I feel much better than before. I have poured out my heart to you (*She showed gratitude with her hand gesture*).	*I sat there, in deep sorrow and anguish with Natasha, compassionate, and feeling the pain of death.*
C12	Thank you for calling me so that I could be with you in your sorrow and pain, all the beloved family members. I feel honored to come alongside your loss and your pain. Is there anything I can do Natasha before I go?	*I felt an emotional connection with Natasha at the loss of her four close family members within four months.*
P12	Please, pray for me and my grieving family. We need the grace of God to comfort us. Pray for God's protection for my family from these mysterious deaths. Prayer for my daughter who was found dead, and we don't even know the cause of	*Silence and presence. I realized the importance of Chaplaincy as I was with Natasha during*

	her death. Pray for my brother's, aunt's, and my mother's souls to rest in eternal peace. I feel peaceful now and thank you for giving me your shoulder to cry on. Chaplaincy helps when your Pastor is far away without access to him in his time of need. *(She bowed her head and closed her eyes as I prayed).*	
C13	Let's pray. *"Our gracious Heavenly God, I pray for Natasha and her family. They have gone through a lot, the four deaths within four months. We continue to trust God and His faithfulness. Be with her even if she is not feeling well with covid. May you to what to do. Give her strength and peace. In Christ's Name. Amen.*	*I felt the presence of God as I prayed with Natasha.*

P14	Thank you, Chaplain Sam, I am so grateful for coming to be with me in this dire situation I have never had in my life. Thank you for your service and your support. Do you have a Bible? I need one. Thank you.	*I was so grateful to be with Natasha in her grief that affected me and made me cry inside.*

C14	You are welcome. Yes. I will bring it, shortly. Thank you for allowing me to be with you in your space of grief.	.
P15	Be blessed always!	

C15	Thank you! (*Then I left the room*)	

Reason for Visit: The patient is in response to the Telmediq page.

Assessment: **of** **spiritual** **needs/resources:** Patient communicated spiritual distress related to peace.

Needs:
Natasha said she feels overwhelmed with social and relational circumstances that are contributing to overall stress. She shared feelings of pain and grief over all the losses they have suffered with the death of important persons in their lives, her mother, her aunt, her brother, and her daughter within a short period. She said that she wrestles with finding peace about that. She requested a prayer for her family who are still grieving for the four deaths and her speedy recovery as she said she has Covid-19 and pneumonia. Natasha asked for a Bible as well. She was emotional as she spoke about the death of her aunt, her mother, her brother, and her daughter who was found dead in the house.

Strengths:

Natasha engaged in self-reflection, and reporters can ask for help and are willing to accept it when offered. She shared a connection with God that supports her ability to cope. She described their family as very caring and supportive, which patients say helps them to have hope. Natasha reported that she is a Christian and that she has 8 children, 4 biological children, and 4 adopted children, including 18 grandchildren. She reported they have regular practices, including prayer that gives hope.

Intervention:

- Explored sources of peace/comfort to help find peace.
- Identified relationship strengths to equip the patient for positive coping.
- Used the patient's faith tradition (Christian, Pentecostal) to ease spiritual distress.

- Provided prayer and a Bible to provide solidarity in grief/comfort.

Next Steps/Follow-up: Spiritual needs addressed, consult complete. The spiritual care team remains available for additional support as needed.

Dr. Rev. Sam S. Mhlanga: (Chaplain Resident). D.Ed., M.Ed., M.Th., M.Div., PhD (cand).

VI.   REFLECTION ON THE VISIT

7.   EQ, emotional self-awareness

I felt sad to hear Natasha's anguish for her four beloved family members, including his mother and daughter. I felt sad, frustrated, and emotionally connected with Natasha's grief as I have grieved my sister recently who died, and my mother who died in 2019. I was aware of Natasha's emotions and feelings and what she was going through.

EQ, awareness of others' emotions

I was aware of the emotions of Natasha and her grief, mourning the four members of her family.

8.   At which points did you feel connected/disconnected?

I felt connected with Natasha as a Christian and at her grief because I also grieved my sister this year, 2022. I did not feel disconnected from Natasha.

a.   What strategy of disconnection did you use?

9.   What were your strengths?

My strengths were action, reflection, and action with Natasha about her four deaths in her family and coming alongside her in her grief.

10.   What did you struggle with?

I struggled to desist from advising and teaching Natasha.

11.   State what you would do differently during the visit by listing specifically in the dialogue where and what you might have done. As you look at alternative relational stances, do you have any insights about what caused you to take a particular stance, and why now would you choose something different?

I would do differently by listening to more of her emotions and reflecting without too much probing but by asking her open-ended or generative questions.

12.   What factors in your personal history, culture, or family system may have influenced your assessment and response to this situation?   Did the encounter remind you of anyone/ any situation in your life? How might this have impacted on the visit?

I come from Zimbabwe in Africa and my personal history, culture, and family systems, as well as my faith background, have influenced me in my assessments and responses to different situations. However, having lived in the USA for 15 years, I have learned about American culture in my assessment too.

13.   **Spiritual Assessment of patient/family:** (the sentence from your chart notes)

8.   Based on your assessment what did you do? (Intervention – describe what you did in the encounter)

Intervention:

- Explored sources of peace/comfort to help find peace.
- Identified relationship strengths to equip the patient for positive coping.
- Used the patient's faith tradition (Christian) to ease spiritual distress.
- Provided prayer and a Bible to provide solidarity in grief/comfort.

9.   What did you learn about your pastoral role and function?

I learned that deep listening, coming alongside the patients in their difficult situations, and understanding my personal feelings and those of my patients are the foundation of pastoral role and function. I have learned to embrace every religion of my patients without any biases.

10.   What learning goals did you work on during this visit? I believe I worked on three of my goals on this visit.

1. My first goal is to name my emotions and those of patients.

2. My second goal is to reflect on patients' feelings and to ask generative questions, open-ended questions.

3. My third goal is to be open and willing to learn and reflect on patients' stories and their past experiences.

11.   What Level I/II outcomes did you work on?
Level II.

12.   Describe the learning needs you identified from this visit.
I need to listen more, understand my emotions and those of my patients more, and come alongside them in an empathetic way. Not to ask questions but to listen and reflect on the patient's emotions and ask generative questions and open-ended questions.

13.   Theological Reflection
What sacred or archetypal story or image comes up for you as you reflect on this visit?

The image that comes up in my mind is King David, mourning the death of his son. When his son died, he stopped fasting and praying and began to eat as he exclaimed that his son was not coming back to life on earth but that he would join him in heaven.

14.   Write a prayer or mindful or heartfelt thoughts for your patient and another for yourself.

Lord, may you comfort Natasha and the rest of her family during this difficult time. Give her peace, strength, and comfort. Please, Lord, give her your Spirit and peace, to endure this difficult time. Amen.

VERBATIM III EXAMPLE

I.   DATA ABOUT CPE STUDENT AND PATIENT

CPE Student:
My name is Sam S. Mhlanga, and I am originally from Zimbabwe in Southern Africa. My denomination is the Southern Baptist Convention. I am an African in my fifties and I am married to Judith, and we have five children.

Patient's name: Carol
Carol is 62 years old, and she is a female Caucasian. She is married and has five children with her husband. She is Bahai.

Date Visited patient/family:
Length of Visit: 45 minutes

Staff Consultations: Before I saw the patient, I checked with the nurse who told me about the patient's condition and how she was processing her diagnosis. When I entered Carol's room, I was aware of what she was going through, emotionally. The nurse had debriefed me about the patient's condition.

Medical Diagnosis: Carol has a history of Ehlers-Danlos syndrome, chronic MAC, asthma, GERD, Diabetes, Heart problems, and Liver damage. (Smoker, alcoholism).

Reason for presenting this visit: I am bringing this verbatim to show how to learn to connect with a patient of a different faith.

My three goals:

4. **My first goal is to understand my emotions and those of patients.**

I will continue to have this goal with the purpose of improving my understanding of my emotions and those of patients. I plan to fulfill this goal by listening with my heart to patients' emotions.

5. **My second goal is to reflect on patients' feelings and not to question them.**

I will fulfill this goal by intentionally, putting on the mindset, repeating it in my mind when I enter patients' rooms, "Reflection, Reflection, Reflection", "Not being inquisitive."

6. **My third goal is to be open and willing to learn and reflect on patients' stories and their past experiences.**

I intend to fulfill this goal by intentionally, thick-listening patients' stories and their past experiences, showing them with facial expressions and nodding to encourage and to show them that I am interested in their stories.

II.   OBSERVATION AND AWARENESS

E.   First impressions and observations: The door was closed, the patient was lying on her bed the room was clean, and her room was overlooking a beautiful view of the river. I was impressed by the cleanliness of the room of Carol. She was sitting on the bed with a cheerful outlook and a happy smile.

F. EQ - Awareness of self before visit: I was not aware of what I was going to encounter because it was routine rounds on my 6th floor, but I was prepared to meet any patient regardless of her condition. However, when I checked with the nurse, she debriefed me about the patient's condition and spiritual needs.

III. SPIRITUAL CARE ENCOUNTER WITH THE LIVING HUMAN DOCUMENT:

Please identify the speakers; for example: C=Chaplain, P=Patient

speaker	Dialogue, spoken and non-verbal	Internal experience – feelings/thoughts/self-awareness
C1	(*The door was closed*) Knock, knock. My name is Chaplain Sam, one of the Chaplains at Tacoma Hospital. Are you Carol?	*I was checking to see if she was Carol and if she would allow me into her room.*
P1	Yes. My name is Carol. (*Smiling*)	*I asked if I could sit on the chair beside the patient's bed, and my eyes were focused on her.*
C2	How are you doing, Carol, today? (*She seemed to be not in*	*I was imagining how Carol was coping with all the diagnoses of heart,*

		pain, but she was very lively and more energetic).	*liver, diabetes, Ehlers-Danlos syndrome, chronic MAC, asthma, and GERD.*
P2		Thank you, Chaplain Sam, for coming. I do not even know how I am living with such kinds of illnesses. But I am trying to be strong for my family.	*I empathized with Carol and what she was going through.*
C3		It sounds like you are going through a lot in your life, Carol. *(I was checking with her how she was feeling and her emotions about the multiple diseases she has.*	*I felt for Carol for her sicknesses because there are several diagnoses she has.*
P3		Chaplain Sam, I am a Bahai, and my religion keeps me going through a lot. My husband and I have five children. I joined this religion because of my husband. I have found meaning in life because of the Bahai faith. However, I am still being inflicted with all these kinds because of the evil in the world.	*The empathy gripped me for Carol. I had compassion and sympathy for Carol. I was touched by her illness, and I resonated with Carol's situation and connected it with my close sister, Stabile, who died in April this year because of some infection on her wound after she broke her leg. The world is full of mysteries of life.*

C4	I can imagine how much you are going through. It sounds like you are going through a lot, Carol.	
P4	Yes, I am distressed because of these diseases but I don't show it to people. My husband and my children are incredibly supportive.	*Carol looked well and fit by merely looking at her, ever smiling with a cheerful outlook.*
C5	Carol, it sounds like you are going through some emotions, I can see you tearing up.	*I was trying to affirm what she was showing with her tears streaming down her cheeks.*
P5	Yes, it is distressing. I have been given dietary meals to eat, accordingly. But so far, I eat through this bag of water that has all the food nutrients going into my bloodstream. I feel sad and frustrated about this dietary plan I must follow. (*Shading tears*).	*I was silent, listening with my heart and waiting for her to finish crying.*

| C6 | It sounds like it is difficult to bear all the sicknesses that you are going through, and you are frustrated with the dietary plan that you must go through daily, especially when you have been | *I was affirming and reiterating what she was telling me.* |

	discharged. The medication that you are to follow daily to keep your body well-balanced.	
P6	I mentioned earlier to you that my faith is rooted in the Bahai faith, and it has kept me going. In the Bahai faith, we have three obligatory prayers: 1. Short Obligatory Prayer. 2. Medium Obligatory Prayer 3. Long Obligatory Prayer.	*As she was talking, I was practicing thick listening, trying to understand her emotions and my emotions too, to connect with her pain. I was trying to understand her faith too because I had never encountered a patient with Bahai faith.*
C7	It's my first time hearing about this religion. I am interested to hear more about it briefly if you don't mind.	*Honestly, I did not know about this religion. When I was doing research, I discovered that it is a religion that emanated from Muslims, from Iran in the 19th century.*
P7	Chaplain Sam, thank you for your interest. Bahai faith teaches that all peoples and religions will unite into one. We believe in the oneness of humanity and the pursuit of world peace. Lastly, we believe in the abolition of all forms of prejudice, the extremes of	*I was applying thick listening as Carol was explaining her religion and how it has helped her during her illness. I was eager to learn how her religion has helped her in her journey of recovery.*

	wealth and poverty. It was founded in the 19th century.	
C8	It sounds like the Bahai religion means a lot to you and your family and how it has helped you to persevere in your illness.	*I was empathic to Carol's health challenges in her family.*
P8	Yes, it means the world to me. All human beings are one.	*My presence was valuable to Carol.*
C9	I hear you, Carol. I resonate with you because my son got so much sick in his early life.	*I was coming alongside and listening to Carol with my heart as she narrated her connection with her faith.*

P9	Chaplain Sam, my faith has kept me moving forward and I don't understand those people without faith what they do when they are facing some challenges in life.	*I nodded my head, cogitating on her condition and worry, imagining how the pain and the feelings she was going through.*
C10	Well, I do not know how they make it without faith in God. I resonate with your imagination, Carol. It sounds like your faith means a lot to you even during this time while you are in the hospital.	*I reflected on her emotions and feelings.*

P10	Yes, it means a lot to me. Thank you for listening to my predicaments and my health challenges.	*I felt compassionate and empathetic to Carol and her family.*
C11	I thank you, Carol, for allowing me to hear about your health challenges and allowing me to listen and to get to know your family. Hope God will give you the strength to pull through this. Is there anything I can do before I leave, Carol?	*I said that while standing up and coming closer to her bed.*
P11	Yes, Chaplain Sam. Please, I need a prayer. I will pray in our Short Obligatory Prayer, and you will close in your way of praying. Sounds good?	*I stood there, thick-listening, compassionate, understanding my feelings and those of Carol, with great empathy. I was excited to hear how she prays according to the Bahai faith.*
C12	Sure. You may start and she extended her hand to me to hold her while we prayed.	*It was comforting to show her my care and to demonstrate that I was there to support her.*
P12	*Mighty God, the God of the universe. I pray that you may bring peace to this world and show us your power. I believe*	*Carol's prayer was short and precise, addressed to God.*

	that people and religions will unite for your sake.	
C13	Let's pray. *"Our gracious Heavenly Father, God, we come to you in humble adoration. I pray for Carol's health now, who is going through health challenges. You know where she is hurting. Touch her soul, her body, her emotions, her inner being, and bring her comfort, and peace that surpasses human understanding. I pray for Carol's family, her husband, the children, and her friends. Please, give them comfort and peace. We pray for all this in the name of our Lord. Amen.*	*I felt the presence of God.*

P14	Thank you, Chaplain Sam, for coming to see me. I appreciate it so much.	*I felt the peace soothing my heart after a prayer.*
C14	You are welcome. Thank you too for your openness. Have a wonderful day!	.
P15	Have a good day too! Bye for now!	

C15	Thank you! (*Then I exited*).	

Reason for Visit: The Chaplain follows up per the spiritual care plan.

Assessment: **of spiritual needs/resources:** Patient communicated spiritual distress related to peace.

Needs:
The patient said feels overwhelmed with various diagnoses that she has and multiple diseases that she is facing which are contributing to overall stress. The patient shared that she is experiencing one disease after another which requires a change of diet and lifestyle for the good of her health. The patient said that she wrestles with finding peace about that sometimes. The patient requested prayer for her holistic recovery, physically and spiritually, and for her family.

Strengths:
Patients are engaged in self-reflection, and reports can ask for help and are willing to accept it when offered. The patient shared a connection with God that supports their ability to cope. The patient described their family as very caring and supportive which the patient says helps them to have hope, especially her spouse, John, and her four children and other family members. Carol is a pleasant patient. Patients reported they have regular practices, including prayer which gives hope.

Intervention:

- Affirmed positive coping strategies to anchor patience in spiritual practices for hope.
- Used the patient's faith tradition (Bahai) to ease spiritual distress.
- Provided prayer to provide solidarity in grief/comfort/encourage the patient.

Next Steps/Follow-up: Spiritual needs addressed, consult complete. The spiritual care team remains available for additional support as needed.

Dr. Rev. Sam S. Mhlanga: (Chaplain Resident). D.Ed., M.Ed., M.Th., M.Div., PhD (cand).

Spiritual Care Team remains available for additional support as needed:

VI.   REFLECTION ON THE VISIT

14.   EQ, emotional self-awareness
I felt sad when I met with Carol and heard about her health issues, and multiple diagnoses. I was aware of the deep grief that Carol was having, and I was aware of Carol's emotions and that affected my emotions too. I have been having many of my family members who were diagnosed with various diseases. I was now aware of what Carol shared with me about what her family was going through with her illness.

15.   EQ, awareness of others' emotions
I was aware of the emotions of Carol when she shared with me that she was diagnosed with multiple diseases.

16.   At which points did you feel connected/disconnected?
I did not feel disconnected from Carol.

I felt connected with Carol emotionally when she told me that she was fine with me praying in my faith and for her to pray in her faith.

a.   What strategy of disconnection did you use?

17.   What were your strengths?
My strengths were action, reflection, and action with Carol about her multiple diagnoses coming alongside her in her sickness, and empathizing with her.

18.   What did you struggle with?
I struggled to avoid advising and teaching.

19.   State what you would do differently during the visit by listing specifically in the dialogue where and what you might have done. As you look at alternative relational stances, do you have any insights about what caused you to take a particular stance, and why now would you choose something different?

I would do differently by listening and reflecting on Carol's emotions and feelings, deeply without asking questions.

20. What factors in your personal history, culture, or family system may have influenced your assessment and response to this situation? Did the encounter remind you of anyone/ any situation in your life? How might this have impacted on the visit?

I come from Zimbabwe and my personal history, culture, and family systems have influenced me in my assessment and response to situations although the American culture has taken over to influence my assessments. It reminded me of my sister, Sithabile Gasela Ncube who passed away in April this year after a short illness.

21. **Spiritual Assessment of patient/family:** (the sentence from your chart notes)

15. Based on your assessment what did you do? (Intervention – describe what you did in the encounter)

Intervention:

- Affirmed positive coping strategies to anchor patience in spiritual practices for hope.
- Used the patient's faith tradition (Bahai) to ease spiritual distress.
- Provided prayer to provide solidarity in grief/comfort/encourage the patient.

16. What did you learn about your pastoral role and function?

I learned that listening, coming alongside the patients in their difficult situations, and understanding my personal feelings and those of my patients are the foundation of pastoral roles and functions. I have learned to embrace every religion of my patients without any biases.

17.   What learning goals did you work on during this visit? I believe I worked on three of my goals on this visit.

- **My first goal is to understand my emotions and those of patients.**

- **My second goal is to learn and reflect on patients' feelings and not to question them.**

- **My third goal is to be open and willing to learn and reflect on patients' stories and their past experiences.**

18.   What Level I/II outcomes did you work on?
Level II.

19.   Describe the learning needs you identified from this visit.
I need to listen more, understand my emotions and those of my patients more, and come alongside them in an empathetic way. Not to ask questions but to listen and reflect on the patient's emotions.

20.   Theological Reflection
What sacred or archetypal story or image comes up for you as you reflect on this visit?

The image that comes up is ten lepers in the Bible who had asked Jesus to heal them.

21.   Write a prayer or mindful or heartfelt thoughts for your patient and another for yourself.

Lord, may you give Carol and the family peace, strength, and comfort to manage, emotionally and physically. Please, Lord, give them your Spirit and peace, to endure this difficult time. Amen.

VERBATIM IV EXAMPLE

Title of this Verbatim: "The Art of Thick-Listening"

I.   DATA ABOUT CPE STUDENT AND PATIENT

CPE Student:
My name is Sam S. Mhlanga, and I am originally from Zimbabwe in Southern Africa. My denomination is the Southern Baptist Convention. I am an African in my fifties and I am married to Judith with five children.

Patient's name Dorothy:
Dorothy is 84 years old, and she is a female Caucasian. She was married but her husband died a few years ago. She is Lutheran.

Date Visited patient/family:
Length of Visit: 20 minutes

Staff Consultations: Before I saw the patient, I checked with the nurse for the patient, and she told me about the patient's condition and how processing. When I entered Dorothy's room, I was now aware of what she was going through, emotionally. The nurse debriefed me about the patient.

Medical Diagnosis: Cancer.

Reason for presenting this visit: I am bringing this verbatim to show how important the art of thick listening is.

My three goals:

1.   **My first goal is to understand my emotions and those of patients and peers.**

2.   **My second goal is to be a thick listener with my heart to both patients and peers.**

3.   **My third goal is to come alongside and understand the feelings of patients and peers.**

II.   OBSERVATION AND AWARENESS

G.   First impressions and observations: The door was opened, and the patient was sitting on the bed the room was clean, and her room overlooked a beautiful view of the river. I was impressed by the cleanliness of the room of Dorothy. She was sitting on the bed with a cheerful outlook and a happy smile.

H.   EQ - Awareness of self before the visit: I was not aware of what I was going to do because it was routine rounds to my 6th floor, but I was prepared to meet any patient regardless of his or her condition. However, when I checked with the nurse, she debriefed me about the patient's condition and spiritual needs.

III. SPIRITUAL CARE ENCOUNTER WITH THE LIVING HUMAN DOCUMENT:

Please identify the speakers; for example: C=Chaplain, P=Patient

speaker	Dialogue, spoken and non-verbal	Internal experience – feelings/thoughts/self-awareness
C1	(*The door was open*) Knock, knock. I am Chaplain Sam, one of the Chaplains at Tacoma Hospital. Are you Dorothy?	*I was checking to see if Dorothy would accept into her room.*
P1	Yes. My name is Dorothy. (*Smiling*)	*I stood beside the patient's bed, and my eyes focused on her.*
C2	How are you doing, Dorothy today? (*She seemed to be in pain, but she was very lively and more energetic*).	*I was imagining how Dorothy was coping with the diagnosis of cancer.*
P2	Thank you, Chaplain Sam, for coming. I have been diagnosed with cancer and I am going	*I empathized with her diagnosis and what she was going through.*

	through distress and downfall. But I am trying to be strong for my two children and grandchildren.	
C3	It sounds like you are going through a difficult period of your life. (*I was trying to check for how long her feelings and emotions about the diagnosis.*	*I felt as if I was a bit pushy and may intrude on her privacy.*
P3	Chaplain Sam, I am a Christian, Lutheran but I am going through a lot. My husband died a few years ago because of cancer. I have a daughter who is going through chemotherapy for breast cancer. My son has also been diagnosed with cancer. Cancer is dancing in my family, and I do not know why going is allowing it to wreck-havoc in my family.	*I felt empathy grip me for Dorothy, and her daughter, Irene. Compassion and love for Dorothy's family touched me and I struggled to understand why God would allow such suffering in this family. I resonated with Dorothy's situation and connected it with my close sister, Sithabile, who died a few days ago because of some infection in her wound. After she broke her leg.*
C4	I can imagine how much you are going through. It sounds like	

	you are through a lot of Dorothy.	
P4	Yes, I am distressed with this disease called cancer. It is running in our bloodstream.	*Dorothy looked tired and distressed and felt for her and her situation.*
C5	I heard you say two of your children have cancer too, how do you feel emotionally?	*I was gently, probing her to hear how she was feeling and checking her emotions.*
P5	I am distressed and I don't know what to do. I feel sad and frustrated because all of us are sick. Who is going to take care of us? (*Shading tears*).	*I took a chair set with her, and I was silent and listening and waiting for her to finish crying.*
C6	It sounds difficult to bear all the sickness that is on you and your children, Dorothy. In the past, when you are faced with such challenges, where do you lean to gain your strength?	*I posed that question to see what kind of spirituality she learns.*
P6	I am a Christian, a Lutheran and I believe in God he is my helper. If it were not God, I would not be here. God gives me strength and I lean on Him.	*As she was talking, I was practicing thick listening to try and understand her emotions and my emotions too, to connect to her pain.*

C7	I am deeply sorry, Dorothy that you are going through such pain and your two children.	
P7	Thank you, chaplain Sam! God is my only hope. I believe in God and my children too are Christians. My husband died a few years ago and it is still fresh for me.	*I was moved emotionally by Dorothy, reflecting on when my mother was sick for a long time and died in 2019. I was applying listening and resonating with her in many ways because I have such illnesses in my family.*
C8	It sounds like the death of your husband affected you a lot.	*I was empathic to Dorothy's health challenges in her family.*
P8	Yes, it affected me and continues to affect me. I am waiting to go and join him in heaven because he was a devoted Christian too. Death is imminent to me.	*My presence was valuable and appreciated as Dorothy narrated how her husband died.*
C9	I hear you, Dorothy. I resonate with you when my family was going through some illnesses and the future seemed oblique.	*As I was coming alongside and listening to Dorothy from my heart, I empathized with Dorothy.*

P9	Chaplain Sam, my daughter is in chemotherapy because of breast cancer, and I am worried about my grandchildren and how they will make it in life.	*I nodded my head, cogitating on her concern and worry, imagining the pain and the feelings she was going through.*
C10	Your daughter is in chemotherapy, she has breast cancer, and you are worried about the future of your grandchildren. It sounds like you are going through a lot, emotionally.	*I reflected on her emotions and feelings.*
P10	Thank you for listening to my predicaments and my health challenges.	*I felt compassionate and empathetic to Dorothy and her family.*
C11	I thank you, Dorothy, for allowing me to hear about your health challenges and allowing me to know your family. Again, I am so sorry that you are going through a lot. Hope God will give you the strength to pull through this. Is there anything I can do before I leave, Dorothy?	*I said that while standing up and coming closer to her bed.*
P11	Yes, Chaplain Sam please, pray for my daughter who is going through chemotherapy, and my	*I stood there, thick-listening, compassionate,*

	grandchildren, my son, and of course for me for God to do His will.	*understanding my feelings and those of the patient, with great empathy.*
C12	Sure. May I hold your hand while we pray?	*I wanted to show love and care and to demonstrate that we are in there to support her.*
P12	Thank you, hold my hand, please!	*My heart was aching for her.*
C13	Let us pray. "Our gracious Heavenly Father. *"Our gracious Heavenly Father, God, we come to you in humble adoration. I pray for Dorothy now, who is going through health. You know where she is hurting. Touch her soul, her body, her emotions, her inner being, and bring her comfort, and peace that supersedes human understanding. I pray for Dorothy's daughter, Sarah who has breast cancer, her son, John who has cancer, and her grandchildren. Please, give them comfort and peace. We pray all this in the name of our Lord, Jesus Christ. Amen.*	*I felt the presence of God.*

P14	Thank you, Chaplain Sam, for seeing me. I appreciate it so much.	*I felt the peace soothing my heart after a prayer.*
C14	You are welcome. Thank you too for your openness. Bye!	.
P15	Have a good day! Bye for now!	

C15	Thank you! (*Then I exited*).	*I wanted to continue to pray for this family because separating from Dorothy seemed to be hard. They could not let him go.*

Reason for Visit: Saw patient on routine rounds.

Assessment: **of spiritual needs/resources:** Patient expressed spiritual coping through Christian faith and supportive relationships.

Needs:

The patient said feels overwhelmed with the diagnosis of cancer which is contributing to overall stress. The patient reported that her daughter has breast cancer too. The patient said that she wrestles with finding peace about that. The patient requested a prayer for her speedy recovery and her daughter.

Strengths:

Patients are engaged in self-reflection, and reports can ask for help and are willing to accept it when offered. The patient shared a connection with God that supports the ability to cope. The patient described their family as very caring and supportive, which the patient says helps them to have hope, especially her daughter Sarah, and her son, John.

Intervention:

- Used the patient's faith tradition (Lutheran) to ease spiritual distress.

- Provided prayer to provide solidarity in grief/comfort and encouraged patient.

- Affirmed positive practices to ease spiritual distress.

Next Steps/Follow-up: Spiritual needs addressed, consult complete. The spiritual care team remains available for additional support as needed.

Dr. Rev. Sam S. Mhlanga: (Chaplain Resident). D.Ed., M.Ed., M.Th., M.Div., PhD (cand).

Spiritual Care Team remains available for additional support as needed:

VI. REFLECTION ON THE VISIT

22. EQ, emotional self-awareness
I felt sad when I met Dorothy and heard about her health issues and cancer diagnosis. I was aware of the deep grief of Dorothy, and I was aware of how Dorothy's emotions could affect my emotions. I have been having many of my family members being diagnosed with every disease and I was aware that what Dorothy shared with me about family cancer, may hurt me hard.

23. EQ, awareness of others' emotions
I was aware of her emotions toward Dorothy when she shared with me that she was diagnosed with cancer, including her daughter, her son, and her late husband.

24. At which points did you feel connected/disconnected?

I felt disconnected with Dorothy when she mentioned that she was mentioned that her death was imminent as if she knew that she would die soon.

- I felt connected with Dorothy emotionally, she told me that she was a Christian because our belief systems are the same. Dorothy talking about God and His sovereignty connected us and praying with her was the point of more connections.

a.   What strategy of disconnection did you use?
I used the strategy of connection, disconnection, and reconnection to check my connection with Dorothy, emotionally.

25.   What were your strengths?
My strengths were reflecting with Dorothy about her cancer diagnosis coming alongside her in her sickness and empathizing with her.

26.   What did you struggle with?
I struggled to avoid advising, teaching, and preaching Dorothy.

27.   State what you would do differently during the visit by listing specifically in the dialogue where and what you might have done. As you look at alternative relational stances, do you have any insights about what caused you to take a particular stance, and why now would you choose something different?

I would do differently by listening and reflecting on Dorothy's emotions and feelings, deeply.

28. What factors in your personal history, culture, or family system may have influenced your assessment and response to this situation? Did the encounter remind you of anyone/ any situation in your life? How might this have impacted on the visit?

I come from Zimbabwe and my personal history, culture, and family systems have influenced me in my assessment and response to situations although the American culture is influenced. The encounter reminded me of my sister, Sithabile Gasela Ncube who passed away last week.

29. **Spiritual Assessment of patient/family:** (the sentence from your chart notes)

22. Based on your assessment what did you do? (Intervention – describe what you did in the encounter)

Intervention:

- Used the patient's faith tradition (Lutheran) to ease spiritual distress.

- Provided prayer to provide solidarity in grief/comfort and encouraged patient.

- Affirmed positive practices to ease spiritual distress.

23. What did you learn about your pastoral role and function?

I learned that listening, coming alongside the patients in their situations, and understanding my personal feelings and those of my patients are the foundation of pastoral roles and functions.

24.   What learning goals did you work on during this visit? I worked on three of my goals during this visit.

- **My first goal is to understand my emotions and those of patients and peers.**

- **My second goal is to be a thick listener with my heart to both patients and peers.**

- **My third goal is to come alongside and understand the emotions of patients and peers.**

25.   What Level I/II outcomes did you work on?
Level II.

26.   Describe the learning needs you identified from this visit.
I need to listen more, understand the emotions of myself and those of my patients more, and come alongside them in an empathetic way.

27.   Theological Reflection
What sacred or archetypal story or image comes up for you as you reflect on this visit?

The image that comes up girl in the Bible who had died, and Jesus raised her from death.

28.　Write a prayer or mindful or heartfelt thoughts for your patient and another for yourself.

Lord, may you give Dorothy and the family peace, strength, and comfort to go through the pain, emotionally and physically, especially, Dorothy and her two children who also have cancer. Please, Lord, give them your Spirit and peace, to endure this challenging time. Amen.

STORY THEOLOGY

During the program of Clinical Pastoral Education, the students are required to author a story theology that captures the essence of connecting them with a personal story that affected them in one way or the other in their career. I chose to write about my son's illness which affected me for the rest of my life. This is the story.

In 2004, our son, Blessing was attending a pre-school when one day, he came from school saying he had seen something that was scary at school, and he could not exactly tell us what it was. He was behaving strangely. We tried to investigate and trace his illness but there was no concrete narrative from the teacher. This illness crushed me and my wife, emotionally. Blessing was five years old, and he became extremely sick, his health deteriorated gradually, from that time. We took him to private hospitals to be evaluated with all forms of technological equipment available. After a few weeks, Blessing developed pneumonia-like symptoms and a high fever. We got scared with my wife of his condition. I was doing evangelism outreach with Rev. Pardon when my wife called me and told me that our son, Blessing, was not feeling well and that had a high body temperature. It was in the middle of the night when she called. I got up and drove back home at night, to Harare. I was incredibly sad to hear that and questioned why it had happened while I was doing His work.

When I arrived, he was extremely sick, and we took him to the hospital, they evaluated his blood to determine any infection in his blood and body. They assessed him for malaria, flu, and many tests but all the tests came back negative. They transferred him to another smaller hospital, but his temperature was always high, and they did not know what kind of infection he had. The hospital where he transferred to was having children who were dying in substantial numbers, and we decided to transfer him to another nearby hospital. I was scared for his life and became emotionally drained with anxiety and anxiety about what would happen to him. When he got to the new hospital, they decided to take him more tests and even a brain scan. When the tests did not indicate any results of any infection, they decided to take spinal fluid samples, and lumbar puncture, which is needed to evaluate the fluid around the brain and spinal cord. The test was to find out if Blessing had meningitis which is a serious infection around the brain. Meningitis may be suspected in babies, but it is usually conducted in babies less than one-month-old. However, they made the test procedure on Blessing. The symptoms of meningitis include vomiting, headache, tiredness, fever, and Blessing exhibited those symptoms. After going through lumbar puncture procedures, Blessing's situation became worse. He could not walk, or speak, and his limbs stifled. He was five years old, and he became like a two-year-old boy. He could not produce any sound, he could not crawl, or do anything. I felt helpless, hopeless, and inadequate as a Pastor and a leader and vulnerable as a leader. My son returned to being a baby again. He was diagnosed with pneumonia, called encephalitis pneumonia (inflammation of the brain) due to infection. The infection is due to infection caused by bacteria or viruses. They confessed that they had made a mistake during the procedure of taking the lumbar puncture tests that caused severe damage to his spine. My trust in doctors was dwindling. I blamed myself for not being home when he got sick. I blamed my wife thinking that she may have exposed my son to cold. I struggled to understand the meaning of all that. We stayed in the hospital with him for more than three weeks.

Our son paralyzed the whole body at our watch. During that time all our three children got the fever too, Blessing, Shalom, and Prosper. However, the other two recovered, and Blessing continued to be sick without any signs of recovery. My wife spent the nights at home with the children and I spent the nights with Blessing at the hospital. Our other children were still young, and they needed much care. We had a housekeeper called Chennai who was a significant help during the day, taking care of the children to help my wife. The sickness of my son affected me grossly and I was refusing even to eat. I was not fasting, but I was not having any appetite to eat anything. My son was only able to eat liquids like yogurt, porridge, etc. He became so skinny that you could see the ribs on his side. During the nights, I would lift him to go to the toilet/bathroom and he was not able to stand on his own or to walk. The Doctors gave up on him and said he would never recover because his brain had inflamed because of the infection. One of the doctors told us that Blessing would never walk, talk, or do anything because his brain had reversed to be that of a two-year-old boy. She said that he would never recover and that we had to take him home because there was no hope in any kind of medication that was available. That statement from one of the doctors crushed my heart and soul. She recommended that we take him to a therapist to help his limbs stretch.

One night, as I saw my son's health deteriorating and his strength gradually and slowly dissipating, I cried to the Lord bitterly beside Blessing's bed at midnight in the Hospital and I asked God why he allowed me to be the Vice Bishop and the Church Administrator of the denomination only to humiliate us by losing our son in His presence. I was blaming God like Adam and Eve. I cried the whole night and begged God to heal my son. After that deep and fervent prayer that night, and complaint to God, I felt God had heard my cry and I felt at peace from that time on, I knew that God would heal my son gradually because He heard my cry and plea. I had a conviction that whatever would take place from now on then, God was in it. However, I felt I had reached the bottom pit, helpless, hopeless, vulnerable, and inadequate.

As the Vice Bishop, one of my duties was to organize and chair the Annual Revival Meetings. I had drafted the programs, planned accordingly, and was prepared to go to the Annual Revival Meetings at Biriri Mission School. It was my job description and mandate to chair the Annual Revival Meeting of more than three thousand attendees. When the sickness struck my son, Blessing, I couldn't go, leaving my son to die of this weird sickness. However, I respect and honor my wife Judith, who encouraged me to go to the meeting saying, that God would take care of the situation. Against all odds, I listened to my wife, Judith, and braced to go to the Annual Revival Meeting in August 2004. However, my heart was pumping whenever I thought of my sick son and my wife, watching over him. By faith I headed to Biriri, leaving my wife with an ailing son and three children.

The Annual Revival Meeting started very well as I chaired the whole meeting and announced that my son was extremely sick to the point of death but that I had to come to fulfill my duty as the chairperson of the event, for God's sake. The members of the church prayed for my son. The Revival Meetings started on Tuesday to Sunday. On Thursday, the whole assembly prayed and some of the people fasted for Blessing, our son to be healed. On Friday, the following day, I called my wife to check how Blessing was doing, and she was happy to tell me that Blessing had started to try to speak, and he was able to say "mama." I reported to the conference and there was a thunderous praise to God from the attendees. There was a progression of his recovery. On Saturday when I called to check his condition again, my wife told me that Blessing was able to crawl and to stand on his own and sometimes hold on tables and chairs. We serve a miracle-working God, indeed! On Sunday, when I went back home, I found Blessing looking alive and recovering well. Within a week, he was able to eat solid food, able to walk, and say some meaningful words. A five-year-old boy who was able to do everything like any five-year-old would do but he had taken three years steps back and now he was recovering right in our watch while we had seen him being struck by paralysis. God is faithful and dependable!

Blessing, spasmodically, recovered slowly but surely. There were certain things that if one were not aware, one would be surprised how a five-year-old could behave in a certain way. Some of the teachers at schools, even though they were informed how Blessing was affected by encephalitis pneumonia, could not understand his situation. His capabilities and abilities were affected, and he needed more time to recover slowly and a lot of support and love. Some of his decisions were, of course, not accurate. When I reflect on my son's sickness, I feel I did not support my wife enough and I regret blaming her and the doctors who tried to save my son's life, and of course for blaming God who healed him.

This event affected me emotionally and still holds a special place in my heart to value every human being's life and health with respect and dignity. When I reflect on the sickness of my son, Blessing, when I visit patients, I empathize and feel their pain. The illness of my son, Blessing, what he went through has changed my perspectives on how I look at sick people and how I treat people who are in critical condition. The experience with my son's predicament forged my attitude toward patients and the way I look at them, treat them, and respect them. I am still struggling emotionally, when I see patients who are struggling to survive, in palliative care and on comfort measures. I am still struggling to come to terms with understanding critically ill people. I am still learning how to get along with sick people.

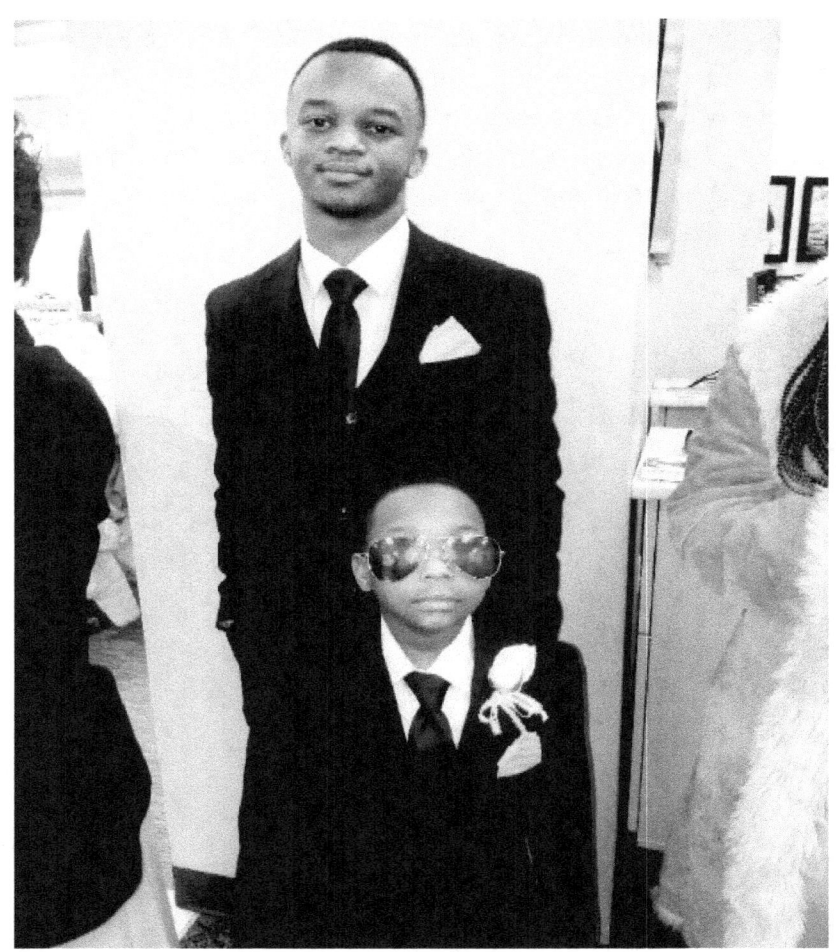

Cultural   Competency   Challenges

Cultural competency is one of the fundamental heartbeats of clinical professional psychology for which every practitioner should be aware, confront, and learn to love it without which failure will be looming. As we now live in a global village, every practitioner will meet diverse patients/clients whom he/she is not familiar with their cultures, customs, norms, religions, belief systems, ethics, and of course, their educational backgrounds hence the importance of culturally competent. Society's diversity and the progressive development of individuals, families, and societies will compel clinical professional psychologists to be more tolerant and patient with other cultures that they have never lived with or among. The challenges of cultural shock should be regarded as strengths and not as weaknesses. Ethnocultural groups that professional practitioners are working with need to be understood in their contexts. "The balance may be achieved elegantly using cultural adaptation procedures. We define cultural adaptation as the systematic modification of an evidence-based treatment (EBT) or intervention protocol to consider language, culture, and context in such a way that it is compatible with the client's cultural patterns, meanings, and values," Bernal, G., Jiménez-Chafey, M. I., & Domenech-Rodrígues, M. M. (2009). P. 261. "An evidence-based cultural adaptation has the potential to provide a methodology to modify treatments systematically so that the culture and context of diverse groups are considered," Ibid. p. 361.

Given that background, I find myself in a challenge when working with a group of people with whom I am not familiar. However, I have worked with various and diverse groups of people which may reduce my ability to collaborate with them, ethically and competently. My challenge will be collaborating with Asian Americans. Their culture and belief systems, values, and languages, do not match with African culture. The fact that they did not colonize Africa unlike the European imperialists, makes us disconnect with the Asians. Europeans and Westerners mingled with Africans during slavery, colonialism, and thereafter when they imposed their cultures, values, and their thinking patterns. Africans can collaborate better with White people because of their historical backgrounds. After the end of slavery, Whites and Black people were forced to live together although they were some intense racism and discrimination. The Union measures such as the Confiscation Acts and Emancipation Proclamation in 1863, the war ended slavery. The Thirteenth Amendment in December 1865 became a legal institution in the USA. Wikipedia, (n.d.). Retrieved November 6, 2018, from https//en.m. Wikipedia.org/wiki/Slavery in the United States.

Therefore, the two groups of people, Black people and Whites were forced to live together in harmony although it did not happen till this day. However, both groups recognize their differences, but they understand each other better. The Asians and Black people have never had such exposure. Therefore, the biases and attitudes between the Black people and the Asians are ridiculously huge. Asians tend to despise the Africans more than what the Whites do. They regard Africans as inferior to them and they love to align with the Whites more. That is why it is rare to see marriages between an African and an Asian.

Cultural competence will be a challenge to have Asians as my clients/patients because of that background. Their values, cultures, attitudes, and biases and my values, culture, attitudes, and biases will hamper my ability to work ethically and competently in my professional practice. However, I will try to minimize the biases by being culturally respectful, loving, and kind and developing good relationships with them. "The delivery of ethical and culturally consistent therapeutic approaches has continued to challenge practitioners today because of demographic changes throughout the country, professional mandates, and the complex manner in which culture is understood and manifested therapeutically," Gallardo, M. E., Johnson, J., Parham, T. A., & Carter, J. A. (2009). p. 246. This will be one of my greatest challenges to foster cultural competence in my clinical professional practice in collaborating with Asians. Applied psychology is still challenged in adequately translating our theories and discourse around multicultural issues into practice. Ibid.

Final Self-Evaluation-Level II

Introduce yourself: My name is Dr. Sam S. Mhlanga, and I am married to Judith, I have five children, four boys, and one girl.

Description of my Clinical Placement Site:

My clinical assignment is Tacoma General Hospital, also covering Mary Bridge Hospital and Allenmore Hospital. At Tacoma General Hospital, I am assigned to the sixth floor. I hold the pager on Mondays and Wednesdays for all four hospitals from 8:00 am to 9:30 am but I hold the pager at Tacoma from 8:00 am to 4:00 pm on Mondays and Wednesdays. Then on Mondays, I hold a pager for TGH, and MBH from 8:00 am to 4:00 pm. On Wednesdays and Fridays, I hold a pager for my sixth floor.

Learning Goals: List your learning goals for the unit and evaluate your progress on each goal.

My Goals:

My first goal is to name my emotions and those of my patients and peers.

I visited a patient who was going through some tough decisions about her medical plan. The patient reported that her illness was terminal, and she knew that she must be put on CMO and said that they would be discussing her final decision with her husband. The patient sounded extremely low in spirits, and I reflected on what she was telling me about her distress and despair.

I sat beside her bed and listened, empathized with her in her situation, and came alongside her. I resonated with her as I remembered my friend whom we used together as College Librarians, and he was diagnosed with lung cancer. He died in a few months as he was preparing for a wedding with his fiancée. It was the painful death of my friend. I felt so sad when I heard the story of Wendy. When Wendy expressed that she was in distress about her diagnosis of terminal illness, I empathized, and I understood her pain because I have friends who have gone through this experience.

I was able to name my emotions when I also visited one of my patients, Frank, who had expressed that he felt isolated and dejected by the family after decades without seeing them. I resonated with Frank in his isolation when I was removed from my family after my father had died at the age of 5 years old and I was sent with my sister to live with my uncle about five hundred miles away from home. I could feel and empathize with Frank, feeling sad and isolated with his family, especially his daughter, Joyce and I was emotionally attached to his situation as I experienced the same.

My second goal is to be a thick listener with my heart to both patients and peers.

While I was visiting a patient on my routine rounds, I checked with the staff nurse about the patient before I went in. The staff nurse broke down, becoming emotional, and asked if we could talk. We went to the staff lounge, and he began to pour out his heart, about what he was going through at his home with his son whom he said engaged in neighbor gangs and he did not know what to do. He pointed out that it was so dangerous for him to be involved in the gang because he could be shot by police or the opposite gangsters. He reported that he has repeatedly warned him to desist from joining the group but that he does not listen. He asked me what he could do to help his son get out of that group and contrate to his school.

I acknowledged and affirmed his feelings as a parent. I applied thick listening, understood his emotions, and listened with my heart. I explored with him to understand his relationship with his son. I reflected with him about his son's behavior and how it was affecting him. I entered the emotions when I resonated with him when one of my sons had a similar situation in which he had friends who came to pick him up and drop him off at any time. I had warned him and encouraged him to concentrate on his school, and not hang around with friends who were not concerned with school. I felt sad and mad when I heard him talk from his heart. I am still working on this goal.

This goal is to enhance my skills in reflecting on the patient's feelings and asking my patients generative questions or open-ended questions. This comes as I want to improve by reflecting on the patient's feelings. Reflecting on a patient's feelings is a deeper way of understanding how the patients present their feelings about their situation. To put it into the right perspective, I visited a patient who was having multiple diagnoses, and I took time to understand how she was feeling and coping with the disease. Open-ended questions were explored like it sounds like your faith in Bahai keeps you moving forward with confidence and optimism. May you tell me more about your feelings when you first learned about your diagnosis? I hear you say your husband has been your strength and a pillar in your journey with the diagnosis. I felt sad about her diagnosis.

My third goal is to come alongside and understand the emotions of patients and peers.

I had a patient at Tacoma General Hospital who had been hospitalized because of a car accident that hit him. As a result of the accident, the patient sustained a head injury; his brain was bleeding, and his arms, had broken ribs, and legs. The car hit him on the right side of his body and all his right side was broken. I visited him and he was in a coma, not able to blink, or move, and the doctor said that he would not be able to be conscious again. The family, on the contrary, declared that he would be conscious and believed in the miracle. The father of the patient had agreed with the doctor that he was willing to let go because he did not want his son to suffer for so long. However, the patient's siblings, a brother and a sister thought otherwise. They argued that their brother would be conscious. So, there was a division in the family. Dr. Zenzo called for a meeting of the family, the social worker, a surgeon, and me. The proposed meeting by Dr. Zenzo was suspended because the family was divided and wanted to agree first on the next steps.

After a day, I received the Telmediq, from Dr. Zenzo, calling us for the family meeting as the family had agreed and they were ready. We got into the conference room and Dr. Zenzo updated the family on the patient's condition. Present in the room was Dr. Zenzo, social worker, surgeon, patient's father, Martin, and his wife, three siblings of the patient. The surgeon explained to the family that the patient had a 50 percent chance of surviving. The patient's father reported that when he visited his son, Enock, he opened his eyes when he called him by name and said that he wanted to wake up. The father had now decided to side with his other three children not to pull off the plugs and wait for Enock's recovery. My presence was to listen and observe how the conservation was leading and support the consensus. I sat there attentively, applying thick listening and coming alongside the family. Gary wanted me to experience family meetings and how they concluded about their loved ones. I am growing in this area, and I am still struggling to keep silent as my pastoral experience is to give advice. This is a learning curve for me and growing in this area of thick listening. This week, in this case, I observed how family can be divided on deciding whether to pull the plug on their loved one who was terminally ill or decide to live on supportive machines. The family, unanimously, agreed to let Enock continue in life support machines until nature took him.

Another scenario about fulfilling my third goal is to be open-minded and willing to learn and reflect on a patient's story as a story theology to be able to listen and trace their stories to deduce their connections, their pain, their emotions, and anxieties. A good example to apply my goal is when I visited a patient who told me about his story that shaped his life, perception, and belief system of himself. Brian told me that he grew up being mocked by his peers, and even by his family members because of the shape of his head which is long and big, a kind of deformity. He told me that he grew up believing that he was ugly, worthless, and unwanted in society as many people told him. He said that he developed a self-image of himself, which was awkward, with self-pity and poor self-esteem. Brian said that until he met a Pastor of a kind who told him that he was fearfully and wonderfully, created in the image of God like everyone. He said the Pastor told him that he has the same potential just like any other human being. Brian said that his paradigm of himself changed instantly. He said that he became confident in himself and never listened to anyone who told him otherwise.

The story theology of Brian resonated with me growing up in my uncle's household in which I was despised and mocked by my cousins and my peers that I was not educated. It all changed when I became determined to pursue my education when the opportunity availed itself. I am emotionally attached to B.'s story, which also shaped his life, perception, and belief system of himself and his destiny.

Future Goals

1. To be relational with my students in approach education. I am going to be working at the Center for Theology and Missions as a Professor. I will use Relation Cultural Theory as a model to connect with students and staff.

2. To show my emotions with students, patients, and staff without holding them back. I will start my new job at Sea Mars Clinics as an "Integration Specialist."

3. To be able to balance academics and emotions to connect with others and myself.

ACPE Outcomes of CPE Level II:

To fulfill the outcomes of CPE Level II, L2.1 of my role as a chaplain, I demonstrated pastoral care when I visited a patient who was going through emotional trauma after losing his five-year-old son, because of liver cancer. The father did not want to eat for some days and questioned God why and said it was better for him to die than his son. I came alongside Jerry with his wife, Betty, consoling them with the words of comfort from their Bible as they were Christian. I read them Psalms 22 and 23, per their request, and I was available to them as they mourned their baby. I resonated with them as one of my sisters lost her daughter at the youthful age of 3 years because she was bitten by a snake while sleeping in a hut.

The factors foundational in my ministry/pastoral call, formation, and practice were articulate when I realized how I interact and relate with my peers, certified educator, and the staff in the Hospitals where I was a resident. I became aware of the strengths and limits of my personhood in the ministry when I did not fulfill my duties, missing patients who needed spiritual care. I can now hold on to my faith in a non-imposing manner which happened when I visited a patient who had a different faith, Hindu, and was able to connect and synchronize with him without imposing my faith.

On August 5, 2022, I visited a patient on the fourth floor after the nurse purged Spiritual Care to support a family who's loved one was dying because of pancreatic cancer. The patient was a twenty-five-year-old female. They were Buddhists and from Vietnam by descent. I was honored to support them as a diverse people as we have cultural differences and different races and religions. I researched before I visited them about the resources and prayers they use when loved ones are sick and dying. I used their meditation poem and words of comfort. They were so happy that I was able to get into their shoes to provide emotional support and prayers in their ways. That made us connect and I did not impose my perspectives or my religion. It was so good to be in pity with them and provide spiritual and emotional support in the religion. They appreciated the support.

I was aware of personal, cultural, and pastoral interactions during this visit with the patient. I remained open and engaged with the patient's father and family. I was able to manage "prejudice" in a positive and pastoral manner and brought connection and solidarity.

I demonstrated pastoral skills, including listening and empathic listening when I met a charge nurse, Peter, who said that he was in distress because of his son whom he said his son Aaron was hanging around with dangerous gangsters in his neighborhood. He said that he had warned him several times to desist from playing and befriending the boys who were committing crimes. He said that he was scared for him that he would be harmed or shot. I listened deeply with empathic reflection with Peter as he narrated his frustration about his son who was slipping away towards hanging with the bad guys in the neighborhood. I applied pastoral skills by empathic listening saying, "It sounds like you are not happy with your son's decision to hang around with the bad guys in your neighborhood." Spiritual care and moral support were provided to Peter, and I also resonated with him as one of my sons did a similar thing, hanging out with unpleasant boys in the neighborhood.

I managed a conflict and brought it to a peaceful ending between myself and one of the preceptors. Although the conflict was not a major one, we were able to resolve the conflict amicably. I used clarifying questions to understand the nature of the conflict, acknowledged where I might have errored, and indicated where the preceptor might have errored too. We resolved the issue, reconciled, and reconnected. I have learned to be an effective thick listener although I am still a growing edge.

Assessing patients' strengths and needs is realizing their potential in their religions, belief systems, skills, talents, and cultural traditions. I was visiting patients when the Nurse Manager on my 6th Floor approached me and asked me if we could clean the patients' rooms. She reported to me that she had noticed and observed and other nurses too that they were in certain rooms that patients were dying whenever they were assigned to those rooms. She requested that we cleanse ritually and pray for those rooms. I consulted with Jim Cornwell, my preceptor. We set the date, the time and drafted an invitation email to all the staff and asked the Nurse Manager to send the emails to her staff to meet on a Friday, and we met with the staff. We performed the rituals. We had water in a vase, and pebbles that the staff dropped in the vase having written the room numbers and the desire to clean the room. We finalized our meeting with prayers not addressed to God or any specific name but in unison. The potential, capacity, and strengths of those served are a powerhouse. The interactions and activities among the staff were amazing, and understanding the behavioral sciences depicts human development among human beings. Human behaviors and relationships are the epitome of cultural theory and paradox theory in which people long for belonging.

I actively engaged the literature of the behavioral sciences and its effect on my theology to inform me about my spiritual care strategies. I am able now to integrate the understanding of behavioral science with my theology in pastoral assessment and care plans for my patients.

Managing ministry and administration functions demands accountability, productivity, self-direction, and clear, accurate professional direction. My preceptor Jim assigned me to the sixth floor which had a mixture of intensive care rooms and those who were recovering from surgeries. Planning daily spiritual care for patients for visits, follow-ups, and the staff's spiritual care. Managing incoming Telmediq and responding to texts of staff within 5 minutes. Epic referrals, Code Blues, and phone calls for hospitals. On August 8, 2022, there was a Telmediq from the staff who wanted the chaplain to come and give spiritual to a patient who was going through distress and mental breakdown because of drug abuse. I spent more than 50 minutes listening and coming alongside her, reflecting with her.

After determining that the patient needed more than spiritual care but psychiatric evaluation and assessment for the patient to get the right therapy. I have learned to have the capacity for self-direction and managing accountability. I take leadership responsibility for my sixth floor for spiritual and emotional support for both patients and staff every day when I am on duty.

I demonstrated a sense of pastoral authority as a minister when I visited a patient who was emotionally drained because her mother, brother, aunt, and daughter had died within four months. The patient needed spiritual care and emotional support. I was emotionally present with her for 55 minutes, reflecting on all the losses she had had while she was in the hospital with Covid. I demonstrated the ability of emotional availability and cultural humility to sustain pastoral relationships with a non-judgmental attitude while maintaining professional boundaries with the patient.

I was taking risks by initiating behavior consistent with my learning goals. I managed to time well, setting a record of being punctual all the time for the entire year except once when my car nearly burnt down. I managed to schedule my PTO effectively and follow the schedule of my classes and clinics, appropriately.

I have utilized peer feedback in group interactions in my verbatims, IPR, and didactics. I was able to dialogue with my peers, certified educators, preceptors, nurse managers, and all the staff in the hospital. There are other days when I was not participating fully in the group for example when my father-in-law died, and my dear sister died in 2022. The interaction with the CEP group brought insights on how to interact with patients, for example, the verbatim that I presented on June 21, 22 about James who had colon cancer and prostate cancer and was going through emotional tornados. After presenting the verbatim, the peers and educator pointed out what I would have posed as generative or open-ended questions to get more information. Their feedback gave me insights to interact with patients which I value to this day.

I initiated consultation with my educator about finding someone to come to teach about Child Grief. She gave me the go-ahead to consult John to come and gave us a didactic about grieving children. John came to present the didactic on August 4th, from 12:00 pm to 1:00 pm. John presented a very touching and educational didactic that will benefit us in our ministries.

My interaction with my peers in the group, the certified educator, and the preceptor during my clinical made me consistent in verbal and emotional involvement.

I used self-reflection for input from others for my personal growth. In developing self-supervision through realistic self-evaluation, I used action/reflection/action models of self-learning. In our CPE peer group, many times we had action/reflection/action and we patients. I have developed new levels of initiative and ownership for positive self-feedback.

I also used the connection, disconnection, and reconnection model, for example, when I disconnected with Hai during the IPR when he had disconnected with me when I had asked Jesse to highlight how they interact with people of diverse cultural backgrounds. Hai thought I was not mindful of the time to ask the question. After my apologies, Hai was able to

My self-supervision happened when I was able to plan for room cleansing with some rituals that the managing nurse had initiated, and I took over to plan for it with the staff. It was successful as both the spiritual care team and nurses, therapists, and CNAs attended and participated in the rituals to pray for those rooms where patients were dying when they were placed in those rooms.

Chapter Six: Relational Approach and Clinical Pastoral Education Summarized

The Relational Approach and Clinical Pastoral Education are the two sides of the same coin, to complement student-faculty relationships. "The key concepts of RCT are best understood in the context of relational movement, which is the process of moving through connections; through disconnections; and back into new, transformative, and enhanced connections with others. Being aware of how all relationships move through these distinct phases is referred to as relational awareness. Acquiring this relational awareness is the first step in developing more sophisticated relational capacities that enable one to identify, deconstruct, and resist disconnections and obstacles to mutual empathy in counseling relationships and the broader culture."[20] CPE is an action/reflection professional educational experience. Clinical Pastoral Education's thrust is to foster pastoral/spiritual care as a vital component in the healing process. "Clinical Pastoral Education (CPE) began in 1925 as a form of theological education that takes place not exclusively in academic classrooms, but also in clinical settings where ministry is being practiced. CPE is offered in many kinds of settings: in hospitals and health care including university, children's, and veterans' facilities; in hospices; in psychiatric and community care facilities; in workplace settings; in geriatric and rehabilitation centers; and congregational and parish-based settings."[21]

[20] Dana L. Comstock, Tonya R. Hammer, Julie Strentzsch, Kristi Cannon, Jacqueline Parsons, and Gustavo, Salazar II, *Journal of Counseling & Development* ■ Summer 2008 ■ Volume 86, (Accessed December 12, 2023).

[21] Ibid.

"The Central Relational Paradox As emphasized throughout this article, RCT theorists have asserted that all individuals have yearnings for connection, belonging, and social inclusion. Despite these yearnings, RCT points out that people commonly demonstrate a paradox in the way they address relational issues in their lives... Although it is noted that all individuals yearn to connect with other people in authentic, mutually empathic ways, feelings of vulnerability, fear, shame, suspicion, and mistrust make movement into connection difficult. Understanding how these relational dynamics are reinforced by social injustices and various forms of cultural oppression complements the culturally competent counselor's knowledge of such issues."[22] In the same vein, Clinical pastoral education (CPE) is a combination of professional education and hands-on experience, providing spiritual care to patients, families, and staff members in multi-faith clinical settings.

There are some basic ethics and exacting standards of conduct from various hospitals and institutions for students of Clinical Pastoral Education (CPE). "It is a violation of confidentiality and hospital protocol to publish information on social computing platforms that is related to patient health information. You may not "blog", "follow" patients online, or "friend or accept friend" requests by patients or their family members. Breach of this standard of professional confidentiality is determined by the hospital management and may result in your immediate termination, and further, may incur civil and criminal penalties."[23] The patients' profiles, confidentialities, identities, addresses, credit cards, bank accounts, family members, and all private information are all prohibited from being compromised. In the relational and

[22] Miller & Stiver, *The Healing Connection, Beacon Press*, (Washington, DC), 1997.

[23] MultiCare Good Samaritan Hospital, (Accessed December 15, 2023).

educational approaches and clinical pastoral education, it all needs deep listening and it requires listening from the heart instead of listening from the mind. Deep listening or thick listening emanates out of silence. Thick or deep listening requires people to listen without responding but to give one's best in listening to a patient as he/she pours out one's heart to be heard not to be told what to do.

The patients, most of the time, yearn to be listened to but sometimes the clinicians want to give advice and tell the patients what to do when they face health, family, and social challenges. Clinical pastoral education stands out to propose the idea of patient-centered as a spiritual care therapy, unlike pastoral or counseling settings in which the Pastor or the counselor have the solutions for the members or the clients, respectively. To talk about ourselves to the patients or the clients and to share our feelings with them is blocking them from sharing their feelings and their stories. Often, the patients or the clients want our silence and attentive listening, undivided attention from the clinical and spiritual providers. "Silence can feel awkward and even uncaring at first. It takes some experience in speaking and listening for people to understand how powerful and appreciative simple silence can be, and how knowing that there will be no questions, comments, or side conversations bolsters the sharing... This silence gives space for everyone to finish listening and to appreciate having been allowed into the recesses of the speaker's life. The sense of intimacy is rich and sacred. When the heart is speaking and the heart is listening, silence becomes fulfilling."[24] Listening is an art that is learned and cherished.

Michael Nichols's argument listening in his book, 'The Lost Art of Listening' asserts that there is three "A" when it comes to

[24] Christine C. Robinson, Alicia Hawkins, UU World Magazine Summer 2012, published by the Unitarian Universalist Association, (Accessed December 22, 2023).

genuine listening, what is most needed is: "Attention-put no barriers, pay attention. Appreciation-appreciate other people's points of view. Affirmation-affirm your understanding. Without some signs of understanding and empathy, the patient starts to doubt if you are listening. Effecting listening is achieved by effective communication."[25] The patient is yearning to be listened to, to be heard, and to be understood. That is the DNA of the clinical and spiritual care profession. The clinician in that specialty must understand what they are signing up for and their expectations on the job.

[25] Michael Nichols, The Lost Art of Listening, (Guilford Publications), 2009.

CONSULTATION WITH THE BOARD
Reason for Seeking Consultation

I am seeking this consultation to be assisted in meeting my level I outcomes. The reason for seeking some help in this consultation is to refine my level I outcomes. I want to succeed in my application to become bored board-certified chaplain and a certified educator. In the outcomes of Level I, I realized that I have some blind spots and some growing edges that need to be refined before I move to Level II outcomes. I sometimes talk too long without giving time for my peers to contribute to my other verbatims. For example, in the second of my four verbatims, I wrote a long verbatim that took more time narrating the verbatims and my peers were not able to give feedback. I have discovered that I sometimes switch on my brain and switch off my feelings and the feelings of others.

Emotional intelligence entails being able to understand self-feelings and the feelings of others. I want to grow in understanding the feelings of others, the patients, the patients, and my feelings to be successful in my clinical and spiritual practice. I have sometimes struggled in these areas. However, I have progressed in the foundational primary focus on self-awareness, self-care, crisis management, copying conflicts, and demonstrating the ability to integrate the concepts of my practice. I have conceptualized my pastoral identity, integrating it my theological, spiritual, and faith heritage into my pastoral ministry. I have learned to use the action/reflection method of education. While I maintain my faith tradition and my theological and ethical values I have learned to respect and honor patients and peers with different faiths and religions.

In the verbatim that I presented on December 21, 2021, I learned that I must align with the patients when they ask questions and then refer them to get the answers to their own faiths/belief systems. I must be alongside with patients. I must empathize, be in the pit with them, listen, be emotionally connected with them, and support them all the way. I have realized that I sometimes stand aloof rather than being with the patients. I sometimes switch off my feelings switch on my brain and stand a distance from my patients. I sometimes use my brain instead of my feelings, maintaining my distance from the patient and standing aloof, instead of standing alongside them and feeling their pain.

I learned that during the class discussion, one of my peers realized that for some reason, I and one of the peers was not actively participating in the discussion about a certain topic. I felt as if it was a confrontation and isolating us. I defended myself and told her how she should have told us in a certain way than to isolate us as if we were not part of the class. During our interpersonal relations, there was a continued feud between me and the above-mentioned peer. The supervisor pursued the discussion of the way we talked.

BIBLIOGRAPHY/REFERENCES

Dana L. Comstock, Tonya R. Hammer, Julie Strentzsch, Kristi Cannon, Jacqueline Parsons, and Gustavo Salazar II, Journal of Counseling & Development, Summer 2008, Volume 86, (Accessed April 7, 2023).

Gildemann, Annette, *Advanced Holistic Healing*, Booknook.biz Publishers, 2020.

Jean Baker Miller Training Institute 2023, (Accessed 10 March 2003).

Jordan, Judith V., and Schwartz, Harriet L., *Radical Empathy in Teaching*, March 2018, (Accessed on July 23, 2022).

Miller & Stiver, *The Healing Connection, Beacon Press*, (Washington, DC), 1997.

MultiCare Good Samaritan Hospital, (Accessed December 15, 2023).

Nichols, Michael, *The Lost Art of Listening*, Guilford Publications, 2009.

Robinson, Christine C., and Hawkins, Alicia, UU World Magazine Summer 2012, published by the Unitarian Universalist Association, (Accessed December 22, 2023).

https://www.oliverianschool.org/why-students-need-relational-learning/, (Accessed June 23, 2023).

https://ucsfspiritualcare.org/history, (Accessed August 3, 2023).

https://www.icpt.edu/what-is-cpe.html, (Accessed August 12, 2023).

https://college.mayo.edu/academics/health-sciences-education/clinical-pastoral-education-residency-minnesota/curriculum/, (Accessed August 21, 2023).

https://www.davidfleenor.org/post/what-is-clinical-pastoral-education, (Accessed September 26, 2023).

https://www.oliverianschool.org/why-students-need-relational-learning/ (Accessed October 6, 2023).

https://www.google.com/search?q=relational+approach+to+education, (Accessed November 10, 2023).

https://www.sciencedirect.com/science/article, (Accessed November 10, 2023).